Bouncing Back *from* Pregnancy

The **BODY** BY **GOD** Plan for Getting Your Body and Life Back After Baby Arrives

Dr. Sheri Lerner

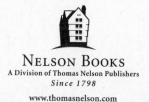

NELSON BOOKS
A Division of Thomas Nelson Publishers
Since 1798
www.thomasnelson.com

Published in Nashville, Tennessee, by Thomas Nelson, Inc.

Nelson Books titles may be purchased in bulk for educational, business, fundraising, or sales promotional use. For information, please e-mail SpecialMarkets@Thomas Nelson.com.

Unless otherwise noted, Scripture quotations are from the *Holy Bible*, NEW LIVING TRANSLATION, copyright © 1996. Used by permission of Tyndale House Publishers, Inc., Wheaton, Illinois 60189. All rights reserved.

Scriptures quotations noted TLB are from THE LIVING BIBLE (Wheaton, Illinois: Tyndale House Publishers, 1971) and are used by permission.

Scriptures quotations noted KJV are from The Holy Bible, KING JAMES VERSION.

Library of Congress Cataloging-in-Publication Data

Lerner, Sheri.
    Bouncing back from pregnancy : the body by god plan for getting your body and life back after baby arrives / Sheri Lerner.
        p. cm.
    ISBN 0-7852-0966-2 (pbk.)
    1. Health—Religious aspects—Christianity. 2. Mothers—Religious life. 3. Physical fitness for women. 4. Mothers—Health and hygiene. 5. Time manage-ment—Religious aspects—Christianity. 6. Lerner, Ben. Body by God. I. Title.
    BT732.L455 2005
    248.8'431—dc22

                                                                        2005008734

Printed in the United States of America

05 06 07 08 09 RRD 9 8 7 6 5 4 3 2 1

I'd like to dedicate this book
to my parents,
Eugene and Diane Schantzenbach

Contents

Part IV: Movement for Bouncing Back

Part V: Stress Management by God for Moms

Part VI: Time Management by God for Moms

The BODY BY GOD
Quick Reference Guide

Your *Body by God Plan for Getting Your Body and Life Back After Baby Arrives* is broken into six sections:

    I. I'm Pregnant. Will I Ever Be Thin Again?
    II. My Baby Is Here! Now What?
    III. Fueling for Bouncing Back
    IV. Movement for Bouncing Back
    V. Stress Management by God for Moms
    VI. Time Management by God for Moms

▶ Important Tip: Start with What's Best for You

If one section of the book interests you more than another right now, you can skip directly to that section.

Together, all of these sections will help you to bounce back after pregnancy effectively and efficiently. As a mother, however, I also realize that there are days when you might need one section more than another, such as the ones on stress or time management.

The following is a quick reference guide to the different areas I will cover. You can start at the beginning and work your way through the book or choose the area that best reflects your needs at the present moment, which will allow you to get immediate answers and results.

▶ Note: Seek Professional Advice

Obviously, in a book this size, we cannot deal with every possible situation that might occur during anyone's pregnancy. Therefore, if you have any questions or concerns at all, please contact your health-care provider.

Where to Turn to See Some Changes Today!

During Pregnancy

Pregnancy can be a wonderful experience, but for many it is filled with challenges. Thankfully, you can do some things to overcome these challenges and make your pregnancy an easier and more enjoyable experience. For help, turn to page 3.

The First Few Weeks After Pregnancy

Sleep deprivation is common for all women with newborns. For some women, postpartum depression sets in as well. The first few weeks can be the most trying, but there is hope. Things *do* get better. I'll show you how on pages 47-60.

Nutrition

To start losing those unwanted pounds you gained during your pregnancy right away, begin adding foods from the Food by God list found on pages 78-81. You will also want to follow the Un-Diet Food Guide found on pages 104-121. This unique guide will help you make remarkable changes in your body.

Exercise

You may now be looking in the mirror and wondering, *Whose body is this?* But you can regain your old figure, and possibly even a better one, by making exercise part of your regular routine. To start, see page 135.

Stress Management

While the words *Mom* and *stress* often seem to go hand in hand, it doesn't have to be that way. All of us—even moms—have the ability to keep stress to a minimum. No, life will never be the same once children enter the picture, but there is good stress *and* bad stress. To live a life without bad stress, turn to page 211.

Time Management

A mother has to be a master of time management. Nothing is more critical to the success of a Body by God family than your ability to manage your time instead of allowing time to manage you. Scheduling time for God, your children, and your spouse will help control stress as well as enhance your life. For help, see page 243.

▶ Caution: Contact Your Health-Care Provider

Before making significant changes in nutritional habits or beginning new forms of exercise, always consult your health-care provider.

Introduction

What's it like to be pregnant? Ask any number of women who have been there and done that, and you'll get almost as many answers. Pregnancy is different for everyone. But God knows *how much* and exactly *what* each of us can handle. Some women never feel better (or more beautiful) than when they are pregnant, while others have a more difficult time. If you're pregnant, remember that God never gives you more than you can deal with, and He intends to go through this pregnancy *with* you, holding your body, soul, and spirit in the palm of His hand. If you've already given birth, it will help you to remember that He will be there for you throughout the days of adjustment ahead as well.

How do I know this? I know it from personal experience, because becoming a mother gave me new insights into my relationship with God. I also know it from Psalm 139:16, which states, "You saw me before I was born and scheduled each day of my life before I began to breathe" (TLB). That's not only true for you, but for your baby as well.

Did you ever wonder if the very first mother, Eve, experienced morning sickness? Remember that she didn't have the benefit of having a mother or friend to talk to about what was happening to her when she began gaining weight and craving ice cream and pickles. She had no one to talk to except Adam, and *he* was in no position to understand how she felt. Eve didn't even have a midwife! (See how blessed *you* are?)

While many things have changed since the day Eve first became pregnant, many things have not. Pregnancy still requires your body to expand and change in ways you never imagined, and you may not like what you see or feel. But keep in mind that these transformations all happen because God has a great gift for you: your child.

Just because your body has altered itself to accommodate your baby, it doesn't have to fall apart and malfunction. God's plan is for you to maintain a healthy body during pregnancy, then bounce back. While not everything will go perfectly—you may not be able to fit into your jeans immediately and may continue to have hormonal breakdowns—you *will* succeed in bouncing back after pregnancy by incorporating God's wisdom into your lifestyle.

Unfortunately, many new mothers put themselves and their health on the back burner due to the demands of motherhood. If you've ever listened to a flight attendant explain how to use an oxygen mask, you know that the first step is to put on your *own* mask, then your child's. The point is the same for new mothers: if you don't take care of yourself first, you won't be able to take care of your child.

As my husband, Dr. Ben Lerner, said in his book, *Body by God: The Owner's Manual for Maximized Living,* by taking time for yourself and following God's Manual for living your life, you will quadruple the time you have for others. You will have more energy and patience, and you will make wiser food, exercise, and time decisions. The long-term results will change both you and your family for the better—both during and after your pregnancy—to make bouncing back easier.

When you look at the photos of me in this book, you'll be tempted to think I've always looked like this and never had issues with my weight. It's not true! At one time in my life I was considered overweight, and I suffered ridicule and humiliation because of it. (I'll explain this at the beginning of Part III of this book: Fueling for Bouncing Back.) Thankfully I was able to change my habits before becoming pregnant with our first child, Nicole. After she was born I could have tried to bounce back *my* way, but instead I chose *God's* way—a healthier, more permanent method. This is what I want to share with you: God's perfect plan to help you to bounce back and maintain a healthy Body by God. It's never too late to begin, so let's start today!

PART I | I'm Pregnant.
Will I Ever Be
Thin Again?

1 | The Body by God in Each Trimester

About a week after I became pregnant, I *knew* it. Even though the pregnancy test results were negative, my instincts were right. My body had already begun to change. For one thing, my breasts were tender immediately. That's a dead giveaway for many.

Thankfully I was healthy and very weight-conscious before I became pregnant. I had been a gymnast for thirteen years, so I was used to checking my weight every day. As an athlete, I was trained to be very attentive to my level of fitness. As a woman, I wanted to look good in my jeans. But as I saw my weight increasing, I feared I was going to feel fat forever, and I experienced an intense emotional struggle. I had great difficulty feeling good about myself.

Eventually I realized I had to set my sights on the end result. The fact that God was about to give me a gift of a child helped me through it, and for that, I knew that I could endure anything. I envisioned myself holding my baby, and in my mind I was fit and trim once again. I tried to keep in mind that my pregnancy, and all that came with it, was part of God's perfect plan for my life.

The First Trimester

For pregnant women, one of two things is going to happen 90 percent of the time: you're either going to be very, very tired, or very, very sick—or both! My first trimester was characterized by a deep fatigue. I had to learn a hard lesson right away: I had to allow myself that extra rest I desperately needed.

When I became pregnant, I had already been a chiropractor for thirteen years. I had a set schedule that worked very well for me. Pregnancy threw this schedule a curveball. My timetable had been pretty much my own to decide, with no one to interrupt or disrupt my life. I was used to rising at five every day in order to spend an hour with God before seeing patients. Soon after I became pregnant, the intense fatigue hit me, and I found I simply could not get out of bed in the morning to keep my appointment with God. I had to allow myself to sleep instead.

I had great difficulty accepting the fact that I needed more sleep than I had ever needed before! Add to that the guilt I felt in putting my physical needs ahead of my commitment to God, and you'll have some idea of the stress I was beginning to feel.

I finally realized that fatigue was part of pregnancy, and God knew all about it. I had to accept the fact that He had given me the responsibility to care for myself as my body nurtured the new life growing within me. That little life was His child, too, and I had to do my best for her! That was my assignment from God for that time in my life. Again, it was for then, not forever (although I *did* suspect my life would never be quite the same again!).

One day He explained it to me so that I could accept the change in my schedule: He had taken my life to a new level, and that necessitated change. He had given me an awesome responsibility, and I didn't need to feel guilty about accepting it. After all, He invented pregnancy in the first place, so He certainly understood what I was experiencing and my body's need for extra rest.

Of all the areas where I could cut back, I knew my personal time with God was not one of them. I needed Him more than ever before! For me, snatches of time spent with God worked well. I began to find minutes to spend with Him while I was working out, walking or running, and in between patients. That time I spent with

Him in the first hours of the day was private and special for me, and I did not want to sacrifice it!

You may have heard of John and Charles Wesley, the founders of the Methodist movement in England during the eighteenth century. Their mother, Susannah Wesley, had seventeen children (yes, seventeen). When she needed time alone with God, there was nowhere she could go to be alone, so she simply sat down wherever she was and threw her apron skirt over her head! When the children saw her with the apron over her head, they knew she was spending time with God and they were not to disturb her. It worked!

Susannah was not only creative about getting time with God, she was also flexible. At the same time, she sacrificed doing other things in order to find that time with Him. She may not have finished the final load of laundry, swept the front porch, or dusted the living room. She made a conscious choice to eliminate one thing for something of more importance to her.

You, too, may find yourself sacrificing time in some areas of your life to make room for other more important areas during this period. It might mean working fewer hours, cleaning the house every other week instead of weekly, or watching less television daily so that you can go to bed an hour earlier than normal to read. You will find that your schedule requires some tweaking and changes during this time.

Once I relaxed about being so regimented in my spirit and schedule and realized that I didn't have to have a set hour's time to talk to God, I discovered a new closeness with Him. My spiritual life became one continual conversation with Him all day long, not just one hour in the morning. It was great!

Even though I seemed to experience just a great deal of fatigue, many of my friends experienced morning sickness and a heightened sense of smell. Smells that they were totally used to suddenly made them run to the bathroom. While there is no cure-all prescription for morning sickness, there are several potential remedies.

First, keep saltines and club soda by your bedside all the time, and eat frequent small meals instead of fewer larger ones. Wristbands designed to prevent seasickness also seem to be helpful. There is a formula made for babies with upset tummies called Gripes Water. This water is safe to use while pregnant and contains ginger, a known natural remedy for helping an upset stomach. Walking and fresh air seem to help the most. If none of these help you, seek the assistance of your health-care provider, who might be able to prescribe an alternative that better suits your personal situation.

 Come to me, all of you who are weary and carry heavy burdens, and I will give you rest.
—Matthew 11:28

The Second Trimester

During my second trimester, I was still experiencing fatigue but had learned some coping skills. Then my body changes started to become very obvious. I remember attending a business conference with my husband when I was six months pregnant. The conference was held on a cruise ship, and the climate was warm. I wanted to go swimming like everyone else, so I pulled on my bathing suit and then looked in the mirror. It wasn't just one mirror; the room was all mirrors! Every wall and even the ceiling were mirrored! To add to the confusion, the light was different from the light in our home, so nothing looked quite right to me.

I hadn't had a bathing suit on in months, and when I saw myself, I was horrified. It ruined my whole trip. I thought that was the way I really looked. Once I arrived at home, I looked in the mirror and got a completely different perspective. It wasn't nearly as bad as it had looked on that ship! I don't know if the problem was in the ship's mirrors or not, but I do know that your perception of how you look is skewed while you're pregnant. I'm happy to tell you, skewed perception will go away (unless you had it before you were pregnant!).

Once I accepted that I didn't look like the whale I saw in the mirror, I began to enjoy my new belly, knowing that there was a magnificent life growing inside of me. The more I focused on the gift God was giving me, and the more I began to feel Nicole move, the more I began to enjoy my pregnancy. No matter what I looked like, I knew it was only temporary. My responsibility was to do everything I could to take care of the baby.

For the first four weeks of my second trimester, I was able to do the same workout I had maintained for the first trimester. At that point I was running twelve miles a day. (Don't beat yourself up! I was a distance runner and a longtime gymnast!) In the fifth week of my second trimester, I cut back my routine dramatically due to my next and biggest challenge: my small bladder. This wasn't a good thing for my workouts! I could run only two or three miles before I had to head back home. It wasn't long before I had to give up running entirely—except to the bathroom every five minutes.

Not running was a big adjustment for me. I also stopped working at my chiropractic office, which was another huge adjustment. This gave me a lot more time to rest, which I needed, but the changes in my schedule were difficult. I knew, however, that it was important that I do the right thing for my health and the health of my baby, and my body was telling me that was it.

Your body will give you signals as to what it needs during this time, but some of those signals might be vague and hard to interpret. This is a time when you need to pay extra attention to how you feel. Many of these *feelings* will be normal, such as if you are tired, you most likely just need rest. Yet anytime that you experience a feeling that is not normal, such as dizziness, a rapid heartbeat, or shortness of breath, stop and examine the possible reason for it. If you can't put your finger on what is causing this reaction, check with your health-care provider. It makes sense to err on the side of caution.

 No One Understands What I'm Going Through!

There's a first time for everything. But for Eve, the first mother, *everything* was a first! Can you imagine how she must have felt when she began to gain weight, her belly started expanding, and her moods began going up and down like a yo-yo? To make it worse, she had absolutely no one to talk to who understood what she was going through. Adam certainly was no help. Eve was the founding member of the first women's club: SPW— the Society of Pregnant Women. She blazed the trail that the rest of us follow.

Only one person understood what Eve was experiencing as she watched her body change to accommodate the new life within her—only one person who could give her advice. Only one person who could truly say, "I know you'll do fine. I'll be right there with you, every step of the way." That was God. When it comes right down to it, it's you and God. The prophet Jeremiah referred to Him as *Elohim Mikarov,* translated "the God who is near" (Jeremiah 23:23 KJV): "Am I a God at hand, saith the LORD, and not a God afar off?" Of course He is! What a comfort!

Because He is God, He knows what a woman experiences when she is pregnant. Because He is God, He cannot break His promise, and He has promised to be near you at all times, whether you think you need Him or not. Who better to watch over that new life growing within you than the God who created it in the first place? Because He is God, you can trust Him to get you through anything and everything that goes along with pregnancy. He knows you love your child already. He loves that baby too. He has provided everything you need, and He will see you through everything to come.

God created Eve perfectly. She had everything she needed to be the world's first mother. He gave her the physical organs to get pregnant and give birth, the stamina to face it all, and the instincts to be a great mother. Did Eve know she had all these resources available to her? How could she, since no one had been through a pregnancy before? She didn't even know what she would need. But God knew, and He provided it for her in advance.

He also provided Eve with a body that would bounce back after the baby arrived. Eve must have worried when her belly began to swell. She must have been shocked at the changes in herself, including the fatigue and morning sickness. Swollen ankles, inability to sleep, back pain, varicose veins—Eve must have hated it all. What kept her going was the knowledge that God had it all planned, and she trusted Him to be with her through it.

While she was waiting for the birth of her baby, Eve had no books to read to learn how to take care of herself. Most likely she maintained her active lifestyle as much as possible, and that helped her feel better. She helped Adam tend their garden, she ate properly, and she walked and enjoyed swimming for exercise. She made sure she took care of herself and the baby growing inside her. She did everything right . . . instinctively.

When Cain was born, no one was more amazed than Eve—except Adam. Remember that no one had ever seen a baby before! Cain was the first one ever born. This was all new ground for the first set of parents, and they both knew they were totally dependent on God for wisdom in raising their child and helping him come to know God. I think that for Eve, holding that beautiful little boy made all the problems of pregnancy disappear from memory, and the joy of having her son made it worth everything she had endured.

—Scripture reference: Genesis 2:18–4:1

▲ ▲ ▲

The Third Trimester

As I entered my third trimester, my small frame began to rapidly gain weight, and my self-image was beginning to warp once again. My attitude toward my body surprised me because when I look at a pregnant woman, I think how wonderfully beautiful she is. I believe most people see a pregnant woman in this light.

Unfortunately, I didn't feel the same way about *my* pregnant body. It was a big challenge for me. Deposits of cellulite that appeared out of nowhere contributed to the poor image I had of my body, and therefore, of myself as a person. Cottage cheese everywhere! Along with this came the aches and pains in my muscles and joints. I knew part of this was because my hips were widening to prepare my body for delivering the baby. Added to this were the frequent bathroom trips, swollen ankles, and more fatigue.

I was tired of being pregnant and ready to go into labor. I prayed that the day would be soon and that God would deliver a healthy child. He did. On February 14, Valentine's Day, Nicole was born.

 ## Chiropractic Care Can Help

I believe that it is extremely important, to both you and your baby, that you receive regular chiropractic care through your entire pregnancy. I don't say that just because I'm a chiropractor. In our practices, both my husband and I have observed the difference it makes with our pregnant patients. The ones who receive regular chiropractic care seem to have easier and quicker deliveries.

For example, I had one patient who came in after the birth of her first child. She had experienced severe sciatic pain while she was pregnant. During the birth she suffered a large vaginal tear and many, many hours of labor in delivery. After the birth, the sciatic pain didn't go away, so she came to me as a patient. She improved dramatically over the period of a year, and then she became pregnant again.

That time, however, she continued her regular chiropractic treatments, and she had no sciatic pain. We all were wondering how the delivery was going to be for her the second time around. Her baby was heavier by one-and-a-half pounds than the first one, and she delivered very quickly and easily—with no tear. Chiropractic care had definitely made a difference, and there are several reasons why.

First, the nerves that control the reproductive system and hormonal balance come from the lower part of the spine. When these nerves are free of interference, the reproductive organs work properly, and they produce the appropriate amount of hormones your body needs to keep you in balance; this will aid in your baby's development.

Second, getting adjusted makes sure that the pelvis is balanced, which allows for proper movement of the fetus. It aids in the baby's ability to turn and allows for easier separation of the pelvis during delivery.

Finally, if your baby is breach, there is a turning technique that is a non-invasive and painless adjustment. I have personally performed this technique on some of my clients and within just a few adjustments, the baby turned.

▲ ▲ ▲

2 | Movement to Make Bouncing Back Easier

When God created man, He created him perfectly and in a manner that allowed him to move in any way he needed to in order to survive. When God was done, man had legs for running and walking, arms for pulling and pushing, and a strong back for lifting and carrying. When God created woman, He created a helper to man who could do all the same things man could to ensure their mutual survival. When God created woman able to bear children, He wasn't about to create a situation that would halt the great gift of movement that He had given her. That would defeat His purpose and possibly adversely affect her survival. Pregnancy requires additional care, including movement.

Our literal survival may no longer be in jeopardy, but not moving could affect the survival of a healthy body. Your health, and the health of your unborn child, as well as the quality of that health, can be adversely affected if you eliminate movement from your life. Not making movement part of your life could make you susceptible to illness, obesity, or gestational diabetes. Therefore it is critical that you continue to incorporate movement into your schedule while pregnant.

Not only is movement important to your health while pregnant, but it also will help you to bounce back more quickly once you give birth. If you have a child already, you know the importance of feeling good, healthy, and fit after your child is born just to keep up with taking care of two instead of one. If this is your first child, trust those who have already been through pregnancy, and realize the importance of movement.

Some women think pregnancy is a time to put their feet up, give their bodies a break, and relax for nine months. I don't think this is what God envisioned for any body for nine months—maybe nine minutes a day or per hour, but certainly not the entire nine months. Movement is as critical to the health of your body, to the health of your unborn child, and to bouncing back after delivery, as oxygen is to your survival.

▶ Word of Caution: Start Smart

If you are starting a fitness regimen while pregnant, you need to be closely supervised. Talk to your health-care provider before beginning any exercise routine.

The Benefits of Movement During Pregnancy

You will find that movement during pregnancy helps you, helps your baby, and helps your body bounce back more quickly, but let's start with how it will help *you*.

Unfortunately, along with the joys of being pregnant and the excitement of a new baby on its way come a lot of possible side effects. Many women experience extreme fatigue, morning sickness, and lack of appetite during the first few months. As your body and baby grow, you may experience your circulation slowing down, which might cause swelling of your hands, ankles, feet, and legs. Pregnancy may also cause leg cramps and varicose veins. The added fat that your body accumulates can cause excessive weight gain or accumulate as cellulite on your hips and thighs. Because your hormones are on the super-duper roller coaster of their lives, mood swings, disrupted sleeping patterns, and depression might set in. There is also the added pressure on your back and spine, causing backaches and subluxation.

(*Subluxation* is a misalignment of your spine that interferes with your nervous system, and unfortunately, there aren't always symptoms. By the time pain becomes a symptom, often the damage is in a more acute phase.) Then, of course, there are always those unmentionables, which we will mention, such as constipation, rectal pressure, and hemorrhoids. Doesn't pregnancy sound fun?

Thankfully, most women do not experience *all* of these symptoms, and their annoyance with those that they do have is minimized because of the expectation of their babies to come. But even if you are the most positive woman in the world, some of these symptoms will bother you at one time or another. That's where movement comes in: it can help eliminate many of these side effects, or make them less annoying.

Movement can:

- decrease fatigue
- increase stamina
- reduce incidences of morning sickness
- help you to sleep
- improve circulation
- result in less swelling of hands, ankles, and legs
- cause fewer leg cramps and varicose veins
- lower body-fat levels
- improve your mood and attitude
- reduce incidences of back pain
- prevent constipation and hemorrhoids
- prevent gestational diabetes

Movement during pregnancy can also create a more enjoyable delivery! That's a funny statement because if there is one thing that *every* delivery isn't—it's enjoyable! But by continuing to move throughout your pregnancy, you will make a positive difference in your actual labor and delivery experience.

Women who exercise during pregnancy tend to have:

- more endurance/less exhaustion during delivery
- fewer Cesarean sections (C-sections)
- fewer episiotomies and epidurals
- fewer delivery complications
- quicker post-labor recovery

The final benefit, however, of movement during pregnancy is the fact that it will help you to *bounce back more quickly!* It only makes sense that when you continue to keep up a level of healthy movement throughout pregnancy, your body will remain fit and healthy, making it *easier* to bounce back. But if you failed to exercise during pregnancy, don't chastise yourself. The key is simply to start.

Who Should Not Exercise During Pregnancy

There will be some women who, for some reason, cannot or should not exercise during pregnancy. As I said previously, check with your medical professional before beginning any exercise program while pregnant. But if you are currently exercising and experience any of the following, please *stop* immediately. Take these warning signs seriously, and seek assistance.

Warning signs include:

- Pain—especially in the abdominal, pelvic, hip, or back areas
- Difficulty breathing
- Spotting or bleeding
- Dizziness or light-headedness
- Rise in temperature
- Sudden swelling in feet, hands, or face

Pay attention to your body. This is a period of time when you need to be more body-cognitive than ever. Warning symptoms are just that—they are warning you that something is not right.

Throughout my pregnancy, I received little warning signals that I chose to ignore. For example, I got very dizzy every time I walked upstairs (and sometimes down), and I had to sit down and put my head between my knees. Never having been pregnant before, I thought it was just another normal side effect and that those episodes would pass. That was an incorrect assumption.

I began my labor and had Nicole at home. Then I struggled to deliver the placenta for four hours. My midwife said there wasn't a lot of bleeding, but it felt just the opposite to me. I finally had to be taken to the hospital to deliver the placenta. When they took my blood pressure at the hospital, it was twenty over twelve! I crashed.

They finally stabilized my body and ran several tests that revealed I was extremely anemic. That explained the dizziness and a few other things as well. If I had listened to my body more and recognized these as warning signs instead of normal pregnancy symptoms, this might have not escalated to the point it did. Therefore I urge you really to pay attention to your body, and seek advice whenever you question anything.

What Movement Is Safe During Pregnancy?

If you are new to exercise, choose some low-impact movement such as walking or swimming. If you are a little more experienced and one who participates regularly in exercise, you might continue with whatever type of activity you currently are doing or add hiking or jogging. The goal is simply to participate in any movement that is comfortable and allows you the most fitness with the maximum amount of safety to your baby. Whatever exercise you choose, the goal is simply to move.

One exception is any exercise where you lie flat on your back on the floor. You should avoid this type of exercise throughout your pregnancy because it decreases blood flow to the uterus.

Swimming and water sports are nice low-impact exercises for you to enjoy. They provide great cardiovascular benefits, and there is little risk of falling or injuring yourself or your baby. You can swim or simply walk in the water. The resistance from the water when walking is great for your legs. Some even use water weights on their legs while walking for a more effective workout.

If you choose walking (which is probably the most universal movement that everyone can easily participate in), you can enjoy doing it outside or on a treadmill in the comfort of your own home. Walking is something all women *should* do unless there is some physical reason that your health-care provider doesn't recommend it for you. The key to making this exercise the most effective for your body is proper heart rate monitoring, which I discuss in detail in Part IV: Movement for Bouncing Back.

For those of you who want to step it up a notch like me, you can run, jog, hike, or use man-made exercise machines such as the elliptical trainer. Just keep in mind that this is not a time to do record-breaking workouts or try strenuous exercises for the first time. No matter what you are doing, stay in your comfort zone, and do not push yourself to new heights. Use common sense.

In fact, pregnancy is most likely a time to cut back. You should also keep in mind that getting too overheated is not a good idea during pregnancy. Even though you have the ability to cool down, it is more difficult for your baby; therefore, especially during the first trimester, moderation is the key.

As I've mentioned, even though I was able to continue my routine of running twelve miles a day during my early pregnancy, it wasn't long before I had to cut it back to under five miles and then eliminate running altogether. Even though I wanted to continue to exercise at my former level, my body could not tolerate it. This didn't mean I had to give up movement entirely, though. That was the time walking became the safest and most effective movement for my body. The key is to listen to your body and make the appropriate adjustments.

No matter what exercise and movement you choose to incorporate into your schedule, you must warm up and stretch before beginning. To warm up, all you need to do is start walking slowly. Increase your speed slightly and continue to walk for a minimum of five minutes. Then stop and stretch for five minutes. Doing this before participating in any exercise or movement will help you avoid injury. During pregnancy, your muscles and ligaments are very supple and elastic. This can make them prone to strains or tears; therefore, take more time than you normally would to warm up. Also, don't forget your water. Drink plenty of water before, during, and after exercising to keep you and your baby hydrated.

Exercises for Easier Delivery

Just as no two pregnancies are exactly the same, neither are any two deliveries. Some women experience relatively easy deliveries, while others have long, difficult labor. No science can exactly determine which you will have before you are due. You'll just have to trust that God will not give you more than you and your body can handle. I certainly questioned that during my twenty hours of difficult labor, but He kept His word, and I did in fact get through it. Getting chiropractic adjustments during delivery also kept my back labor to a minimum.

Kegels are a form of exercise for your vaginal and perineal areas. They strengthen the pelvic-floor muscles. Many women do these exercises so they are less likely to have urine leakage during their third trimester, but many have found that they also help during delivery. Kegels are easy and you can do them any time (while watching television, talking on the phone, or even sitting at a red light). No one will know you are doing them. They are easiest done in a sitting position, but with practice you can also do them standing or walking.

How to Do Kegel Exercises

1. Tighten the muscles of your pelvic floor (between your vagina and anus). *To locate these muscles, act as if you were going to try to stop your urine flow.*
2. Hold this tightened position for approximately ten seconds, and then release.
3. Repeat this exercise ten times.
4. Gradually increase the number of Kegels you do each time and the length of time you hold the contraction.
5. Try to work up to three or four sets a day.

Movements to Avoid During Pregnancy

- Jumping
- Abdominal work
- Exercise that requires you to lie on your back, due to its decreasing blood flow to the uterus
- Actions that could cause loss of balance or falling (i.e., skiing)
- Contact sports where you could get hit
- Movement that causes you to get overheated or dehydrated
- Heavy lifting
- No movement at all, such as long periods of sitting

▶ Note: To Move or Not to Move?

There may be more movements that you should avoid during your pregnancy. Check with your health-care specialist.

Being Health-Conscious Helps

I had to continually remind myself that the weight that piled on could (and *would*) also be worked off *after* the baby arrived. The determined and disciplined health-conscious exercise devotee that I had been for so long, I told myself, would help me through that brief period and back to where I was physically before I became pregnant.

Continuing with my habit of exercise and movement, and keeping my chin up throughout the nine months, was a daily challenge, but I prayed my way through it and worked out as much as I could. The exercise and movement really helped, not only with the physical part of staying as fit as possible, but with the emotional part of feeling better about myself.

Another thing that helped tremendously was having friends who had experienced the same feelings I had. I began to realize that those who had been health-conscious and exercised before their pregnancies eventually did get back into shape after their babies were born. Those who didn't care so much about nutrition and exercise couldn't seem to lose that extra five or ten pounds of baby weight after the birth. This observation convinced me that it was probably possible to get back into shape. (I know one woman who gained one hundred pounds over the term of her pregnancy, and she lost it all after her baby was born.) If you weren't thin before your pregnancy, however, it will be harder to *get* thin after it.

What helped me lose the weight after the birth? Because of my gymnastic training and healthy-eating lifestyle, when I became pregnant, I was in the best shape ever. The weight I gained over the nine months came off with consistent exercise and good eating habits. For you this might not be the case, since not everyone is a gymnast. The point is that movement will help take the weight off after pregnancy. It doesn't matter whether you work or are a stay-at-home mom. Implementing any movement into your schedule will make a difference, whether it is a walk on your lunch break or going to the gym. Don't be discouraged by the size of the task (or the belly): *all* movement *will* help.

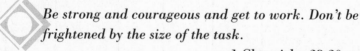

Be strong and courageous and get to work. Don't be frightened by the size of the task.

—1 Chronicles 28:20 TLB

3 | Fueling to Make Bouncing Back Easier

A question that most newly pregnant women ask is: "How much weight should I gain?" Many experts will tell you that you should gain at least twenty-five to thirty-five pounds for a healthy child. If you polled one hundred women, however, you will probably find that they gained anywhere between twenty-five and one hundred pounds! I tried to find some correlation between a woman's original weight and how much she gained, but I couldn't. Some very petite, lightweight women gained twenty-five pounds while others gained a hundred. And the same went for heavier, larger women. The only correlation I could find was that those who exercised and ate well before and during their pregnancies lost the weight (no matter how much it was) more easily than those who did not.

I know that it is virtually impossible not to be weight-conscious during your pregnancy. Your doctor weighs you first thing at each visit, makes a note of it, and then always seems to announce it aloud. All your friends and family seem to want to know month by month how much you've gained, and of course, you are your own worst weight-watcher as you get on the scales each morning to see how much higher the total might be from the day before. The only saving grace is that eventually your belly will be so big, you won't be able to see your toes, let alone the numbers on the scale.

As hard as it might be, this is not a time for watching your weight. It should be a time for watching *what* you eat. It is a time for making good, healthy, Food by God choices for you and your baby.

▶ **Note: Healthy Food Choices**
I detail Food by God and understanding the different types of fuels in full in Part III of this book, beginning on page 67.

Eating for Two

Just because you now have the need to eat for two doesn't mean that you have to double your consumption. Yes, it is important that you increase your diet to include the added calories your baby requires, but that doesn't give you permission to gorge yourself to excess. Most women need an additional three hundred calories per day while pregnant (possibly more if they are exercising), which shouldn't be too difficult to consume. As an example, you might normally eat two thousand calories per day. If you were using the eating-for-two philosophy, you would eat four thousand calories a day! In reality, you would need to consume only twenty-three hundred. So be careful not to buy into the *eating-for-two* mind-set.

▶ **Note: How Many Calories Do You Need?**
Check with your health-care provider for the appropriate number of calories you personally should be consuming.

Then there is the question of what you eat to get the additional three hundred calories you need daily. You could choose a cheeseburger, fries, cake, or cookies, but none of those choices would be the best for you and your growing baby. The best choice, of course, is healthy Food by God packed with the nutrients you and your baby need for maximum health.

Just as overeating is bad for you and your baby, undereating also is not healthy. This is not a time to restrict your eating in any way. Do not diet or try to lose weight during this period. By not eating enough and not getting the appropriate amount of protein, vitamins, and minerals you need, you could harm your baby, causing it to become undernourished or worse. Don't panic, though, if you cannot eat an optimal diet for a few weeks in the beginning of your pregnancy. It happens to the best of us, and your baby will do just fine. If it continues, speak to your health-care provider.

Dealing with Nausea

For those women with a lot of morning sickness, nausea, and heartburn, eating properly in the first few months may be a daunting task. You may also worry that your baby is not getting enough nutrition, but there are some things you can do to help overcome this sick feeling and keep your growing baby properly nourished.

- Eat small meals.
- Eat dry foods such as crackers, dry cereal, or pretzels.
- Eat small meals, but frequently.
- Eat fresh fruits and vegetables.
- Drink plenty of fluids between meals.
- Avoid greasy, fried, fatty, or spicy foods.
- Avoid unpleasant odors.
- Get regular chiropractic care to insure healthy nerve flow to the digestive system.

According to the Mayo Clinic, 70 percent of women experience some morning sickness. Thankfully its severity tends to lessen as time goes on, and by the second trimester, most nauseous feelings will go away. If nausea persists, however, call your health-care provider.

Dealing with Cravings

You've probably heard many stories about pregnant women and their cravings, and if you're pregnant, now you've experienced it firsthand. The funniest, and probably most common, foods associated with cravings are pickles and ice cream, but I've heard everything from chocolate to mashed potatoes to spicy foods. My friend had even more specific cravings—Kentucky Fried Chicken. No, it couldn't be *any* fried chicken. It had to come from this fast-food restaurant.

After the first three months of my pregnancy, I finally had enough energy to be more normal, more like myself. But then my body really started to change. I wanted food that I had never wanted before. I hate to admit it, but I drove twenty minutes to get a cheese steak three times a week! I got *incredible* cravings. My taste in food totally changed.

Of course I also experienced some normal guilt over giving in to the cravings. Then I realized I might as well enjoy it, as long as I gave in to these cravings only once in a while. Everyone understands that a pregnant woman craves weird foods at odd times of the day and night, right? After all, during pregnancy was the only time I'd be able to get away with it! I did, however, make a conscious choice to eat Food by God 90 percent of the time. Whenever I gave in to a craving, I balanced it by making sure I was also eating good food the majority of the time.

I'm not sure if there is a true scientific reason for cravings, or if it is just an excuse to eat things that we might not normally eat. Many experts say that it is your body letting you know that it needs certain nutrients that are in the foods you crave. Just as your copier or printer will let you know when it needs more ink or toner, your body lets you know exactly what it needs and when.

Food cravings are powerful as they urge you to seek out the foods they want you to consume; but they aren't necessarily always unhealthy. There may actually be a reason you crave salt, sugar, or protein. You just need to continue to maintain a balanced, healthy diet during this period as well. That's where Food by God becomes so important. Even when I craved and ate my cheese steaks in the evening, I still ate a healthy lunch to balance it out.

If your craving is a healthy one, listen to your body and comply. If it isn't, find a healthy alternative. Often something with sweet-tasting spices and flavorings, such as anise, cinnamon, peppermint, spearmint, or maple, does the trick.

What Do I Need During Pregnancy?

I have mentioned the term *Food by God* several times now, but what exactly is it? Food by God is what grows and exists in nature—foods that He made. Foods by Man are those that man has created or altered. It's actually quite easy to know the difference. Some examples of Food by God are fruits, vegetables, beans, nuts, seeds, and natural grains. Some examples of Food by Man are sugary cereals, white breads or pasta, and all other processed foods. Food by Man lacks any usable purpose because it is devoid of nutrition or life. Food by God is all life-giving and full of the nutrition that you and your growing baby need.

I go into great detail about the Food by God and fueling in Part III of this book, but I want to give you a quick overview of the principal areas of focus during pregnancy. If after reading this section you want more information, feel free to skip to Part III. For now, listed below are some of the key facts you should know and concentrate on while pregnant.

[God said,] And look! I have given you the seed-bearing plants throughout the earth, and all the fruit trees for your food.

—Genesis 1:29 TLB

Fruits and Vegetables

Fruits and vegetables have a high consistency of water that is packed with high-quality vitamins, minerals, antioxidants, enzymes, and other nutrients. They are also a great source of natural fiber, which aids in digestion. You should eat three or four servings of these per day.

Protein

Most of your body's tissues are made up of protein. This is why it is extremely important for your baby to get enough protein to help build his or her developing cells and tissue.

Best sources: lean meat, fish, poultry, egg whites, beans, nuts, seeds, almond butter (but not necessarily cheese steaks!).

Calcium

Getting enough calcium in your diet ensures that both you and your baby have healthy and strong bones and teeth. If you do not get enough calcium, your baby may have to draw the calcium he or she needs from your own bones, and that's not good. During the last trimester of your pregnancy, your baby's bones are becoming denser and need more calcium.

Best sources: nuts, seaweed and kelp products, sardines, salmon, wheat germ, bran, spinach, broccoli, almond milk, and organic cheese.

Iron

Pregnancy increases your volume of blood by 50 percent, so producing hemoglobin (which carries oxygen to both you and your baby) becomes a very important task for your body during this time. Without iron, hemoglobin production doesn't happen. Without enough iron, you can become anemic. Most expectant mothers need more iron than nonpregnant women because it aids in the development of their babies' red blood cells and carries oxygen to

muscles and helps them function properly. It also reduces suscepti-
bility to stress and disease. Unfortunately, it can also become toxic if
you consume too much; therefore, always seek help from your medical professional to find out how much iron you personally need.

Best sources: lean red meat, leafy greens such as spinach, dried
fruits, nuts, bran, molasses, seaweed, fortified whole grains, seeds,
raisins, and parsley.

Vitamin A

Vitamin A promotes healthy skin, good eyesight, and growing
bones.

Best sources: carrots, pumpkins, sweet potatoes, spinach,
squash, greens, apricots, cantaloupe.

Vitamin B

Vitamin B helps your body to use protein, fat, and carbohydrates effectively. It aids in the formation of red blood cells and helps
to maintain your nervous system.

Best sources: meat such as fish and poultry, beans, nuts, seeds,
dairy foods, wheat germ, whole grains, avocados.

Vitamin C

Vitamin C helps your body use iron and build healthy gums,
teeth, and bones. But because your body cannot store vitamin C, it
is important that you consume satisfactory amounts daily.

Best sources: citrus fruits, broccoli, tomatoes, fortified fruit juices.

Folic Acid (Foliate)

This is another nutrient that you need to take more of during
pregnancy. A 50 percent increase to a total of six hundred micrograms is usually recommended, especially during the first trimester,
when your baby's spinal cord is developing. Healthy nerve and spinal
cord development depend on adequate amounts of folic acid. Folic

acid is very important to your baby's health *before* conception and in the early months of development. It aids in cell division and helps prevent birth defects.

Best sources: green leafy vegetables, dark yellow fruits and vegetables, beans, peas, whole grains, nuts, yeast, lima beans.

RECOMMENDED DAILY DIETARY ALLOWANCES FOR WOMEN
U.S. FOOD AND DRUG ADMINISTRATION—REVISED 1990

(From the Food and Nutrition Board of the National Academy of Sciences / National Research Council)

Female RDA (by age)	19–24	25–50	Pregnant
Calories	2,200	2,200	2,500
Protein (G)	44	44	60
Calcium (mg)	1,200	1,200	1,200
Iron (mg)	5	15	30
Vitamin A (mcg)	800	800	800
Vitamin B_6 (mg)	1.6	1.6	2.2
Vitamin B_{12} (mcg)	2.0	2.0	2.2
Vitamin C (mg)	60	60	70
Folate (mcg)	180	180	400

Fluids

During pregnancy your body has an even greater demand to remain hydrated. Drink six to eight glasses of water a day. Water is always the best choice, but you can drink some unsweetened juice. Avoid caffeinated and sugary beverages.

Carbohydrates

Carbohydrates are your body's main source of energy.

Best sources: whole grain breads and cereals, potatoes, fruits, vegetables.

Fats and Sweets

Everyone needs some fat so that energy can be stored in the body. Limit it, however, to no more than 30 percent of your daily calories.

Foods to Avoid

While most foods in moderation are fine, there are some foods that you should avoid entirely during your pregnancy. Even though alcohol isn't exactly in a food group, you should avoid it completely during pregnancy. No amount is safe during this period. It is probably also wise to avoid caffeine. If you absolutely cannot do without it, limit yourself and switch to decaffeinated products when possible. Keep in mind that caffeine isn't only in coffee, it is in many sodas, chocolate, and tea.

You might also want to avoid raw eggs, raw meats and fish, and products that are not pasteurized. You should not eat certain fish with high levels of mercury, such as swordfish, shark, and mackerel. Even though some of these are Food by God, you should be careful about consuming them raw in order to keep the risk of possible bacteria or food poisoning to a minimum. Your baby is eating what you are eating, and you want him or her to progress and grow as God intended—fully healthy.

▶ Important Note: Seeking a Good Balance

It is important that you maintain a healthy and nutritional diet throughout your pregnancy. If anything prevents you from eating balanced meals or gaining weight properly, seek help from your health-care provider, registered dietitian, or nutritional expert.

4 | Be Gentle with Yourself

While you're pregnant, be really gentle with yourself. I had to learn that it was okay to give myself a break. I had always been a self-starter and a very active and competent woman. I worked hard and typically had my life organized and in control at all times. The words *I can't* and *no* were not in my vocabulary. Yet during my pregnancy I found that I could no longer do it all and keep up the pace to which I was accustomed. It was very difficult for me to learn to say *I can't* during this period, but I knew it was important to my health and the health of my child.

I had always been the go-to person whom everyone could rely on to pull up the slack and take care of things. I was the one who had a nice, tidy schedule where I fit in everything that I, my husband, my practice, and everyone else needed. But I had to come to grips with the fact that I was not Superwoman. Very few can continue their prepregnancy pace. Once I recognized that, I knew that I wasn't alone; I wasn't just a pregnant woman whining about being too tired to handle her responsibilities. I realized that I had to let up a bit and give myself permission to take breaks and slow down my pace of life. This was a huge transition for me, and it required that I be much gentler with myself. This is a time when you, too, must be gentler with yourself.

Looking back, I see now that I should have relied on my husband more. Even when I wasn't working, I thought I should have been able to handle my other daily responsibilities all by myself. He was busy; my job was to grow a healthy baby, and I was going to do it to the very best of my ability—all by myself. (So I thought!) That was the wrong attitude. For one thing, it cut Ben out of some of the preparation he needed for fatherhood.

I could have asked my husband to pick up dinner after work, get the groceries now and then, or run a few errands. Once Nicole was born, I should have asked him to help me during the night. Sleep is the area in which new mothers are the most deprived. I thought that because I was breast-feeding, Ben couldn't help. In reality, I could have pumped one extra feeding during the day so that he could get up at least once during the night to feed Nicole. If this had happened, I wouldn't have been so exhausted during the day. Even a full night's sleep just once a week would have made a huge difference to me and my ability to cope with my responsibilities.

One other area that men should know is important, even though it is difficult to ask for, is encouragement. Whenever Ben complimented me during and after my pregnancy, it meant the world to me. It lifted my spirits, made me feel appreciated, and reminded me that my husband was trying to be supportive and understanding. Tell your husband once how much his encouragement means, and hopefully, he'll remember it now and then. Don't be afraid to ask for help whenever you need it and from wherever you can get it, even if it is just a verbal comment.

Self-Image

Pregnant women tend to fall into two categories: 1) they love everything about being pregnant, including their bigger bodies, and their self-esteem rises; or 2) they have hesitation and doubt about their changing bodies, and their self-esteem falls. Both are perfectly normal, and it is also perfectly normal for you to feel one way one trimester and another the next. For most women, the first trimester is tough simply because they physically don't feel well. The second trimester, they are feeling better and are starting to enjoy finally showing. It's the third trimester when some women look in the mirror and wonder, *Whose body is this?* That is when self-esteem can drop dramatically. During this time, while some women may feel beautiful, just as many others feel very ugly.

My advice is to be as gentle with yourself as you would be to a friend. Even if my best friend had gained one hundred pounds during pregnancy (which some of my friends did) and looked as big as a house (or maybe as if they ate one!), as a friend I would still tell her that she looked beautiful pregnant. I would encourage her to focus on the gift that God was growing inside of her. Most people would do the same. So why is it that we aren't as kind to ourselves? We know pregnancy is only a temporary situation. I had to keep reminding myself of that. During pregnancy, my body was no longer only God's and mine. It was God's, mine, *and* my baby's. With three of us in there, of course I looked different!

Our society is bombarded with images of what women should look like. Most of these images are of sleek, toned, beautiful women. When your body doesn't look like theirs, it's tough to look yourself in the eye and say, "I'm beautiful too." But God *does* see you as a beautiful woman. He sees a woman who is willing to provide a home for one of His children for nine months. What great sacrifice and what great beauty there are in this. Be gentle with yourself, and try to see yourself through God's eyes, not your own.

Worry

It's normal to worry during pregnancy. Most women worry about everything concerning their unborn babies' health, whether they'll be good parents, and whether their bodies will actually bounce back or be stuck in that blimp-like phase forever. But worry has no purpose other than to consume your thoughts and time. While I wouldn't be human if I didn't worry now and then, when I was pregnant I found comfort in God's Word. Once I realized that God was in charge, I relaxed.

> *Don't worry about anything; instead, pray about everything. Tell God what you need, and thank him for all he has done. If you do this, you will experience God's peace, which is far more wonderful than the human mind can understand. His peace will guard your hearts and minds as you live in Christ Jesus.*
>
> —Philippians 4:6–7

Your Body

You need to be the most gentle with your body. Be alert to the signals it gives you. Some signals may be like beacons in the night; for example, you will know when your body needs rest. If so, give it rest. If it needs fluids, give it fluids. If you are having dizzy spells, as I was, pay attention and find out the cause. I've mentioned that sometimes, however, these signals are like small transmissions that we have to listen hard to hear. This is a period when we have to really pay attention. We must treat our bodies with respect and be mindful that they have their limitations. They may be temples of God, but for now, they are also temples for two, so be more gentle than normal.

> *Kind words are like honey—sweet to the soul and healthy for the body.*
>
> —Proverbs 16:24

Easy Does It

Pregnancies are just as individual as the women who experience them. Some things are predictable and happen to everyone. But the way a woman adjusts to her pregnancy is uniquely hers. That's why it's important to be gentle with yourself while your body and mind are adjusting to being pregnant.

In the Old Testament, Hagar was a woman who had a tremendous amount of stress in her life—some of it brought about by her pregnancy. Hagar was personal maid to Sarai, whose husband, Abram, was a wealthy and prominent citizen. Sarai and Hagar had several major arguments over the fact that Hagar was pregnant and Sarai couldn't get pregnant, no matter what she tried. Finally Hagar couldn't take it anymore and ran away.

God met Hagar in the desert, comforted her, and sent her home to Sarai. He reassured Hagar that she would have a son, and he would leave his mark on the world. God knew exactly what Hagar needed to hear, and that's what He told her. He was loving, kind, and gentle with her, and Hagar responded well. He calmed her down, encouraging her to go easy on herself during that difficult period of her life.

A lot has been said about raging hormones during pregnancy, but the under-lying message is valid: give yourself a break. If you do something that seems off-the-wall or out of character, such as crying or getting angry about things that you normally would not, it's okay. Also, if you don't get everything on your list done, move it to the next day's list. Wonder Woman is a mythological character, so don't try to be her. Being pregnant is your number-one priority for nine months. Other things will have to wait their turn.

During pregnancy, Hagar's body wasn't what she was used to. She didn't look the same, and she didn't feel the same. She should have listened to her body and rested when it demanded rest. She probably didn't have enough water with her to keep her (and the baby) properly hydrated. (Water is heavy, and she wouldn't have been able to carry a sufficient supply for her flight into the desert.) Can you imag-ine what Hagar's self-image must have been like after Sarai finished with her? There she was, plodding through the desert sand, trying to get away from her rant-ing and raving mistress, huge belly slowing her exit, and needing a pit stop every few minutes.

Compared to the nonpregnant women around Sarai's compound, Hagar must have felt as big as Sarai's tent! She needed to be reminded that she was not only eating for two, she was doing everything else for two as well: breathing, sleeping, exercising, walking, planning, and praying. She was trying to do it all, all by herself. In His love, God met her where she was, in her time of greatest discouragement, and at the lowest point of her self-esteem. Because He is a loving, gentle Father, He does that—just when we need it most. If He can be that gentle with us, shouldn't we be gentle with ourselves?

—Scripture reference: Genesis 16:1–16

▲ ▲ ▲

5 | Special Nine-Month Plan for Expecting Mothers

Congratulations! You're going to be a mother! This is both an exciting and scary time for you. How you take care of yourself during your pregnancy and how you provide for your growing baby's health should be your primary concerns right now. In addition to feeling overwhelmed with everything you have to learn and do to insure good health for both of you, you have a life apart from the pregnancy that needs attention as well, especially if you have other children. No question about it: pregnancy is a balancing act!

You are the only one who can assure that your growing baby has the nutrients he or she needs to safely arrive in the world. This is not the time to begin experimenting with handfuls of nutritional supplements or new eating plans. (You should always consult your healthcare professional before doing either of these.) As a result, I thought it would be helpful to recap some of the information I've shared, along with adding some new information, in a simple plan. The following will help make your pregnancy a special and healthy time in your life.

Generally Speaking . . .

Months One, Two, and Three (First Trimester)
Fueling
- Start taking a good prenatal vitamin (such as the Body by God Prenatal Vitamins).

- Stay hydrated; drink at least eight glasses of water each day.
- Avoid all alcohol, tobacco, and recreational drugs; and limit, if not eliminate, your caffeine intake.
- Don't take any medication unless your health-care provider approves it.
- Your diet should be high in protein, calcium, and iron.

   a) Protein: Doctors recommend sixty grams of protein per day, which is approximately two servings of protein-rich foods. Good sources are lean meat, fish, poultry, egg whites, beans, nuts, seeds, and almond butter.

   b) Calcium: You should be getting approximately twelve hundred milligrams of calcium per day. The best sources are nuts, seaweed and kelp products, sardines, salmon, wheat germ, bran, spinach, broccoli, and cheese. You may need to take a calcium supplement to meet this requirement.

   c) Iron: Your iron requirement doubles to thirty milligrams per day. Again, you may need to take a supplement to meet this requirement, but good sources are lean red meat, leafy greens such as spinach, dried fruits, nuts, bran, molasses, raisins, seaweed, fortified whole grains, seeds, and parsley.

- Because folic acid is so important the first few months of pregnancy for your growing baby, it is recommended that you take a supplement of four hundred micrograms. Good natural sources for folic acid are green leafy vegetables, dark-yellow fruits and vegetables, beans, peas, whole grains, nuts, yeast, and lima beans.
- Now is not the time to diet. You need to begin adding three hundred calories per day to your diet; however, these extra calories should come from Food by God.
- Because morning sickness may hinder your ability to eat, start eating small but frequent meals. Many women do well on six small meals spaced throughout the day.

- If morning sickness continues to get the best of you, try saltines, club soda, or Gripes Water. (Gripes Water, as I mentioned, is for babies and completely safe during your pregnancy. It contains ginger, which is known for settling the stomach.)

Movement

- If you currently are on an exercise program, continue with it as long as your energy level permits it, but try not to exceed one hour per day.
- If you are *not* currently on an exercise program, check with your health-care provider prior to adding walking, swimming, stretching, yoga, or stationary-bike riding to your schedule. Start slowly and listen to your body; work your way up to thirty minutes three to four times a week.
- There is nothing better for you during this time than walking and fresh air.
- Avoid any heavy lifting, contact sports, jumping, or activities where you could fall.

Stress Management

- Rest as often as you can. Adequate rest can help reduce the incidences of morning sickness, and it will make you feel better and reduce stress.
- Most of the time, your emotions will be running on a roller coaster. Keep in mind, it's not you—it's almost always your hormones when you get upset, down, or stressed.
- Keep in mind that the first three months can be the most tiring, stressful, and difficult. Once past the first trimester, most women start feeling considerably better. If not, consult your health-care provider, but keep your chin up and keep looking forward.

- If you feel stressed about gaining weight, wear a maternity outfit even if you don't need it. Then people will know why you're putting on extra pounds.
- Start a journal. Writing down your feelings will help reduce your stress.
- Connect with other women who are pregnant by joining a pregnancy class.
- Talk to God. It is best to go to Him when stressed.

Time Management
- You may have to cut out some of your routine to gain some resting time. The house doesn't have to be perfectly spotless, with everything in its proper place. Ease up on your household chores if necessary.
- Make phone calls while exercising or resting.
- Review your calendar now, and make appropriate scheduling plans for maternity leave from work (if needed).

Months Four, Five, and Six (Second Trimester)
Fueling
- Continue the fueling recommendations from the first trimester.
- You should begin to feel better and have less morning sickness. You will most likely begin to crave foods. Eat something good prior to giving in to a craving.
- This is a time where you will feel like eating for two. Continue to eat the Foods by God, and try not to consume more than an additional three hundred calories per day.

Movement
- Maintain your movement schedule from the first trimester.
- Discontinue any exercise that requires you to lie on your back or right side. This may restrict blood flow to the baby.

- Begin to wear comfortable, loose clothing. This will not be the time to worry about being the fashion plate you once were. The key is comfort.
- Reevaluate your footwear. Wear comfortable shoes with good support.
- Be conscious of your posture. Stand tall and try not to hunch forward.
- Stop bending over at the waist. Start squatting by bending at the knees when retrieving items low to the ground.

Stress Management
- Continue writing in your journal. This might be a great gift for your child when he or she is older.
- Continue to talk to God, especially when you are stressed. He is *always* there for you. Try to keep in mind these Scriptures: "God is our refuge and strength, a tested help in times of trouble" (Psalm 46:1 TLB); "I advise you, O daughter, not to fret" (Psalm 45:10 TLB); and "I will never, *never* fail you nor forsake you" (Hebrews 13:5 TLB).
- Your belly is starting to pop out, so people can now see that you are pregnant. Relax and enjoy the attention you are getting.
- Take pictures of your growing belly for your baby book.
- Go shopping for maternity clothes, baby furniture, and other baby items.
- Start taking weekly date nights with your husband. Go to dinner or a movie. This will become even more important to reduce stress after the baby is born.
- Spend more time with pregnant friends, or consider joining a pregnancy class. This is a great way to compare symptoms and remedies and vent emotions. Other pregnant women will understand as no one else can.

Time Management
- Your energy level will begin to increase, allowing you to accomplish more.
- Register now at gift registries at local stores.
- Start preparing your baby's space. Ask friends or family or hire someone to do the painting and heavy work.
- Sign up for and schedule classes on childbirth, Lamaze, or breast-feeding now.
- Review your health insurance. If you have questions, get the answers now.

Months Seven, Eight, and Nine (Third Trimester)
Fueling
- Keep up the good work by eating Foods by God.
- Increase your intake of fiber and green leafy vegetables to help avoid constipation and hemorrhoids.
- Increase your fluid intake and decrease your salt intake to help reduce the effects of swelling and water retention.
- Eat fewer spicy and greasy foods to avoid heartburn.
- It may be necessary to eat five to six small meals a day instead of three large meals to aid in digestion.
- Keep in mind that just because your belly is growing more rapidly, you don't have to eat more. Continue with the extra three hundred calories per day.

Movement
- Decrease the intensity of your workouts. For some, this may mean eliminating them except for walking.
- Avoid long periods of sitting, as this will slow circulation.
- Continue to walk to improve your circulation. This will help eliminate swelling of hands, ankles, and legs. It will also reduce occurrences of leg cramps, varicose veins, and lower back pain.

- Continue to be aware of your posture and movements. Try to stand as tall as possible to avoid back pain.
- Put your feet up when needed, and do gentle stretches.
- Begin Kegel exercises to strengthen your pelvic muscles.

Stress Management
- Don't give up date nights with your spouse.
- Have a girls' day off and do something fun with friends.
- Your body is growing more quickly, and your new shape could cause stress. Many women feel more beautiful than ever during this period, while others feel uncomfortable. Focus on your baby, not your shape.
- Consider making a plaster cast of your belly. It will be fun to compare your pregnancy and postpregnancy bodies. It will also encourage you to see how far you've already come in getting your old shape back.
- Anticipation of having a newborn and of being a new mother might be stressing you out. Talk to your husband or friends, and remember that God is vitally concerned with both you and your baby. He will help you.
- Three to four times a day, stop what you are doing and put your feet up and relax.
- Choose baby names.

Time Management
- Continue to buy the things you will need for your baby.
- Buy your baby announcements and address them now. If you are having the announcements printed, compile a list of names and addresses so they are ready to go.
- Finish fixing up your baby's new space.
- Tour your birthing facility, and work out a detailed plan for getting there once you go into labor.

- Make arrangements for the care of your other children while you are in the hospital.
- Make a list of the people and phone numbers to call once the baby is born.
- Pack your hospital bag. Don't forget your camera!

PART II | My Baby Is Here! Now What?

6 | The First Four Weeks with a Newborn

For thirteen years I had been a single, independent working woman. I was used to a schedule where I was responsible only for myself—one person. Then Ben and I got married. This was an adjustment, because then I had two people's schedules to consider. It wasn't too long after I found out I was pregnant that there were three of us.

As soon as Nicole was born, I stopped working to stay home and take care of her. To me, that meant I was no longer working forty hours outside of the house, so I should have been responsible for 100 percent of what went on within the home. I nearly killed myself trying—I'm sure many of you can relate.

Even though I had had a difficult time with delivery and was severely anemic, my self-sufficiency kicked back in as soon as I got home. I was nursing every two hours, which was excruciatingly painful for me, and I wasn't sleeping. I almost drove myself to the point of collapse the first three days Nicole was here.

Because Ben was working at the office, I never wanted to bother him for help when he got home. I believed I should be able to handle it all, and I felt such guilt for not being able to do that. I didn't understand that asking for help did not make me a bad mother.

One night Nicole wasn't sleeping well, and I had been sitting in a chair, holding her for five straight hours, and was at the point of exhaustion myself. Finally I woke Ben up and asked him just to hold her so I could get some sleep. He was glad to do it, and it gave him some precious bonding time with our daughter. This was my first lesson in asking for help.

Thankfully, my mother was able to come down to Florida to help me out on the fourth day. This was great support and relief for me. Still, Nicole never slept through the night until she was seven months old. This was exhausting. When she was four months old, I took another lesson in asking for aid and decided to hire someone to help me out for two hours a day, twice a week. My intention was to use this time to go for a run, but instead I found that I simply crawled back into bed to catch up on my sleep.

Even though I fought against ever asking for help, it's important that you do when you need to. No man (or woman) is an island. We all need support at times.

I realize that not all women will have the advantages I did, especially if you are a single mother or live away from family. This is a good time to accept the help of friends and women in your church. Other mothers have a wealth of experience and will understand what you are going through and what you need. Don't be afraid to ask these people if they know someone who might be able to help, just until you get back on your feet.

Chiropractic care during this period was also lifesaving for me. Because of so many hours of holding Nicole (not to mention my double-D–sized breasts), I developed acute upper back pain. Chiropractic was critical for me and helped me to avoid taking pain medications, which would enter my breast milk.

The first few weeks with Nicole were a time of bonding and learning. Even though so much of motherhood is instinctive, there is still much that you cannot know or understand until you actually experience it. Changing diapers, bathing your baby, and breast-feeding can be instinctive or learned, but the emotional connection and deep sense of love you feel as soon as your baby is placed in your arms cannot be taught or even explained. This one feeling alone made any difficulty I experienced over the previous nine months worth every minute. It also gave me a deeper sense for the love that God has for each and every one of us.

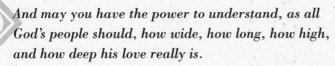

And may you have the power to understand, as all God's people should, how wide, how long, how high, and how deep his love really is.

—Ephesians 3:18

What to Expect After Delivery

If at all possible, you should spend the first four to six weeks after delivery resting when your baby is resting. You will need all of your energy to take care of yourself and your baby. You will also probably experience some vaginal bleeding for six to eight weeks following delivery, which may cause you to become anemic and more tired. This is normal, so don't be alarmed unless the bleeding is excessive (more than you experience with a normal period). Consult your health-care professional.

During this time, your body begins gradually to return to normal. It will take up to six weeks for your uterus to return to its pre-baby size, your cervix to shrink, and your vagina to regain its muscle tone after being stretched during the birthing process. Ovulation, menstruation, and hormones will all return as early as four weeks after the delivery as well.

If you are like most women, your biggest concern at this time will be your abdomen. Right now it looks like an old, wrinkled, deflated beach ball hanging off the front of your body. But don't feel pressure to start doing sit-ups immediately. Many physicians will want you to wait until your six-week checkup before beginning any exercise program. My advice is to listen to your body. As soon as you feel able to begin to return to your normal activities, speak to your health-care specialist. If he or she gives the okay, get started immediately, because the sooner you begin, the sooner you will bounce back.

 Mommy's Little Bundle of Joy

How do you raise the Son of Almighty God? As you would any baby: very carefully, wrapped in prayer. Mary of Nazareth knew her newborn baby boy was God in the flesh, sent to provide a way for people to find their way back to Him. God gave this young teenager an awesome responsibility. She would have been less than normal if she had felt equal to the task.

All new mothers feel out of their depth when it comes to raising a first child. Newborns don't always sleep or eat well. Reading all the literature available for new mothers can sometimes be confusing. What makes up for the sense of inadequacy is the overwhelming love you feel for your baby as you care for him or her. For Mary, however, there was the added responsibility of her little boy being God Himself, in human form. How she must have poured out her heart to God asking for advice!

Nurturing is what mothers do best, and while Mary nurtured her baby, I suspect she took care of herself as well. When He napped, she napped beside Him. When He nursed at her breast, she gently stroked His cheek with her finger. When He fussed at night, she walked around the house, holding Him and singing to Him. And Mary let Joseph support her during her recovery.

Surely Mary's husband, Joseph, was a tremendous help supporting her during her recovery, and he loved the baby as if He were his own son. To give Mary a break, Joseph took Jesus into the carpentry shop with him, settling Him in the beautifully carved wooden cradle he had made for Him during Mary's pregnancy. He wanted the boy to grow up with the sweet smell of sawdust in His nostrils and the soft swish of planing in His ears. Joseph was happy that Mary asked him to help her with the baby because he wanted to be a good daddy.

Having a newborn around the house was a challenge, to be sure, but it was also a rich blessing in their lives. Joseph was pleased that Mary wasn't trying to do it all herself but leaned on him to help wherever he could. While it is safe to say that not all fathers are that attentive and helpful, Joseph was a true help to Mary.

She seemed to be healing nicely from the birth and the arduous trip back to Nazareth from Bethlehem, where they had gone for the government-ordered census around Mary's due date. As a man, Joseph still resented that Mary had to give birth in a stable because all the hotel rooms were full. That was not at all what he had wanted for his wife, but they had managed, with God's help. Joseph hummed softly as the baby gurgled happily in His cradle, and he thanked God for a wife who let him be a big part of this special little boy's life.

We'll never know if Jesus had diaper rash, colic, or any of the other things that a newborn can experience. And we don't need to know. Since God chose Mary, we can presume that Mary was an excellent mother, giving her baby all the loving care and attention He needed to grow into His destiny. From the time Jesus was born until He was twelve years old, the Bible is silent about His life. It's safe to assume He was a normal kid, learning how to function in everyday life. Joseph and Mary taught Him what He needed to know, and as we are told in Luke 2:52, He "increased in wisdom and stature, and in favour with God and man."

—Scripture reference: Luke 2:1–7, 39–52 KJV

▲ ▲ ▲

Breast-Feeding

The first few weeks with a newborn are when you master breast-feeding—or not! No one told me to prepare for this daunting task. Maybe it would have helped, and maybe not. For me, however, breast-feeding was very difficult, and I would have traded it for another twenty hours of hard labor giving birth any day. The first four weeks, I dreaded Nicole's feedings every two hours. My breasts were sore, and my nipples were raw and bloodied. One breast was so bad that I finally couldn't nurse from that side, so I had to pump it. What I pumped ended up looking like pink milk due to my blood-ied nipple.

I felt it would take a miracle to continue like that, and if Ben had suggested I quit, I probably would have considered it—at least for a moment. But I *wouldn't* have considered it for long because I knew the benefits breast-feeding had for my baby, as well as me. I persisted and even consulted with a lactation specialist in the hopes she could help me.

Unfortunately she couldn't help, so I continued, still experiencing pain and discomfort, over the next four months. When Nicole was six months old, I was visiting with friends and nursed in front of them. My friend immediately noticed that Nicole was nursing with her lips tucked in instead of like a fish. As soon as we adjusted her lips, it made nursing much easier, and I had no further problems. I stopped nursing when she was nine months old.

Despite the difficulty I had nursing, I'm glad I did it. Not only was it the healthiest decision for my baby, but also it helped boost my own metabolism to get pounds off and help me bounce back. In fact, the last six months that I breast-fed, I could have eaten desserts for every meal (but I didn't!) and not have gained weight. I actually was thinner than before I was pregnant during that time. Many of my friends experienced the same thing. I believe this is something God has given new mothers to assist in the bouncing-back process. If you don't lose weight while nursing, however, don't worry. As long as you continue to eat a healthy diet and exercise, the weight will come off in time, and you are still doing what is healthiest for you and your baby.

Just because my experience was difficult doesn't mean yours will be. I know many women who do not experience any discomfort and find it very enjoyable. My suggestion is to commit to trying to breast-feed your baby. Do it for as long as you can so that both you and your baby will reap the benefits that God has planned. I'm certain you will be glad you did.

Not everyone, however, will choose to breast-feed, and some cannot nurse for one reason or another. If breast-feeding is not an option for you, don't feel guilty about it. You will simply need to find an alternative. Some women may seek the help of a wet nurse, while others will use pre-made formula. A friend of mine tried to breast-feed, but after four weeks she wasn't able to produce adequate supplies of milk. After researching various formulas, she chose one to replace her breast milk.

If you have the option, even a few weeks of breast milk is very beneficial to your baby. If not, talk to your pediatrician to find a good solution.

Tip: Breast Is Best

What's good for your baby is good for you too!

Benefits of Breast-Feeding for Your Baby

- The first few days of breast-feeding, your milk is actually *colostrum*, which is full of antibodies to help fight infection, bacteria, and viruses.
- Breast milk provides greater protection against common diseases and your baby's ability to fight them off.
- Breast milk is perfectly mixed with the exact amount of nutrients, fat, sugar, water, amino acids, and protein that your baby needs.
- Most babies find breast milk easier to digest.
- A breast-fed baby grows faster initially but then levels off and maintains normal weight levels longer in life. Recent studies at the Mayo Clinic suggest it may protect against obesity later in life.
- Breast-fed babies have lower rates of illnesses such as ear infections, allergies, and other medical problems (see http://medicalreporter.health.org/tmr0297/breast-feed0297.html).
- Breast-fed babies have a lower rate of bottle tooth decay, which typically affects the exterior of the front teeth of the baby—unlike cavities, which can affect all teeth.

- Hand-to-eye coordination is optimized by suckling at a breast (see www.lactationconnection.com).
- Human milk is always sterile. You don't have to worry about preparing bottles and nipples.

Benefits of Breast-Feeding for You

- It provides an emotional bond and closeness to your baby.
- It helps your uterus return to its original size more quickly.
- It delays menstrual cycles.
- It boosts your metabolism.
- It helps you lose weight more rapidly.
- It helps you to sustain your weight loss.
- It makes your baby healthy, and it's less stressful to care for healthy babies.
- It decreases your risk of breast cancer, according to the American Cancer Society (www.cancer.org).
- It decreases your risk of ovarian and uterine cancers.

Again, for those of you who cannot, or choose not to, breast-feed, don't lose heart. You and your baby can still achieve health by following the guidelines for movement and nutrition throughout this book.

Tips for Successful Breast-Feeding

Preparing your nipples (or "roughing them up") prior to birth by scrubbing them with a washcloth daily is no longer recommended. This tends to remove protective matter from your nipples. Instead, learn the proper way to nurse and you shouldn't have difficulties. Seek the assistance of a lactation consultant *before* having your baby. Your health-care provider, whether an OB/GYN or a midwife, should be able to suggest a specialist in your area. If Nicole had been suckling properly, I most likely would not have experienced such difficulty. Breast-feeding should not be painful, and cracked and bleeding nipples are *not* normal. The typical cause of this is simply improper nursing positioning.

This might sound funny to you, but to prevent engorging of your breast, put a chilled cabbage leaf in your bra. Use a leaf only one time. I actually did this and never had a problem with engorgement. Little research has been done on this, but it may simply be that because the leaf is chilled it reduces swelling of the breast; some studies showed that cabbage leaves worked more quickly than ice packs. Besides that, they are more flexible and easier to place inside of a bra than an ice pack.

You will find that you will have the biggest breasts you have ever had in your lifetime. I was huge—bigger than cantaloupes, and none of my tops fit. I had to buy larger sizes just so that the buttons didn't burst. Even though I had lost all the weight I wanted to, it took me two years to get back into my prepregnancy bras.

Speaking of bras, the best tip I have for you is to wear bras with good support, especially when exercising. I wore two sports bras—one over the other one—when I ran. I knew that being well supported is critical to breast health, and it also helps to eliminate sagging in the future!

Many of you will enjoy your new cup size, and many of you will not. What matters most, however, are the benefits to both you and your baby as a result of your decision to breast-feed.

7 | Bouncing Back—Where Do I Begin?

It's easy to be totally consumed with the activity of your baby right now—not just because you want to, but because your baby requires it. Even so, this is a good time to start thinking about bouncing back. For most women, vigorous activity is banned for the next four to six weeks, but that doesn't mean *all* activity! There are things you can do to help prepare for bouncing back more quickly during this time:

- Set Realistic Goals
- Eat Healthy
- Begin Movement

Set Realistic Goals

When Nicole was six weeks old, my girlfriends came over to take me out to dinner. I went to my closet to find something to wear. I had thought I'd be back in all my old clothes by that time but found my selection still very limited. I finally found something, looked in the mirror, and saw this big stomach sticking out. I could have gotten upset, but instead I chose to be gentle with myself. I realized *and accepted* that it was okay. I looked fine for a woman who had just given birth six weeks prior. I could have gotten depressed, but I knew that I was doing the things necessary to bounce back, and if I gave my body a little more time, it would.

Getting back to your prepregnancy weight and size is probably your first and foremost physical goal right now, and you'll accomplish this through the gradual reintroduction of movement into your daily schedule. It won't happen overnight, but it *will* happen. First, however, it is important to state that there are some other goals that may need to take precedence over your weight goal for the first few weeks after delivery.

Make Time for Rest and Relaxation

Rest and relaxation will be hard to achieve during at least the first few weeks, if not the first year! Therefore it is important to make sure adequate rest and relaxation opportunities are high on your priority list. Rest when your baby rests, and relax as time permits. If you have other young children at home, this is a good time to pop a video into the VCR and take a break while your children watch it. If you are a working mom, power naps are perfect during lunch breaks at this time.

Find Personal Time for You

As much as you may want to be with your new baby 24/7, it isn't healthy for you or your child. Finding personal time away from your baby will give you the little breaks you need to be always fresh and appreciative of the time you have together. You can find personal time by enlisting the help of your spouse, a friend, or relative. Possibly it is only for a half-hour a day; then you can choose to give yourself a manicure, go for a walk, or take a nap if needed. It's up to you!

Ask for Help

I've mentioned the fact that for many women, asking for help is very difficult. We feel as if it is a sign of weakness or a sign that we are not fit to handle all of our responsibilities. That is not the case. Asking for help when needed is healthy and is evidence of strength of character. Remember, you are not an island and cannot do everything yourself. Forget your ego, and ask others to help when necessary.

Gradually Work Movement Back into Your Schedule

Start slowly, and don't overdo it. This is a time when you cannot push your body too hard, but you can introduce light and low-impact movement into your day so that you can begin to feel the benefits again of exercise.

Eating Healthy

You have spent the past several months consuming at least three hundred more calories per day than prior to becoming pregnant. If you choose to breast-feed, you will now need to increase that by another two hundred calories per day, resulting in an extra five hundred calories total per day more than your original prepregnancy diet. While this may seem like the time to cut back on your calories dramatically to lose the extra pounds you have put on during pregnancy, it is not—if you are breast-feeding. Dieting too soon can cause a decrease in your milk supply and insufficient nutrients for your baby.

If you choose not to breast-feed, now *is* the time to get back to your prepregnancy diet. It's very easy to continue to eat as much as you were while pregnant. After all, you consumed more food every day for the past nine months, which most likely created a new habit. Breaking this habit may be a bit difficult, but your motivation to regain your body shape will help.

Another thing that is difficult during this period is your new time schedule. Because you are up in the middle of the night for feedings, your body will often say to you, "I'm awake. It has been several hours since I last ate. Feed me!" Even though I was very strict about my diet and nutrition, when I was up in the middle of the night feeding my baby, I wanted a snack too. I felt I deserved it for being up! I seemed to navigate toward the ice cream and cookies most nights, but then I used some creative thinking to come up with a few healthy snacks such as raisins or celery with almond butter.

The key is simply to eat a well-balanced and nutritious diet full of fresh fruits, vegetables, and whole grains and other Food by God until this, too, becomes a habit.

Beginning Movement

Your movement is going to depend on your level of fitness and your recuperation from your delivery. Typically you can resume *some* low-impact activity, such as walking, one to two weeks after a vaginal birth. If you had a Cesarean birth, you will probably have to wait three to four weeks. Six weeks is ordinarily the wait for any running or high-impact activities.

I took short walks starting the week following Nicole's birth. Because I was so anemic, I really had to take it easy. If I went for a walk, that meant I didn't have the energy to go grocery shopping that day. If I really needed groceries, the walk had to wait. There was a lot of compromise during that period.

Your movement should be tailored to your own needs and abilities, but during this period it will be pretty limited. Don't be too hard on yourself for not jumping right back into your prebaby exercise routine. During the first couple of weeks, moving at all will be difficult while you deal with episiotomy or Cesarian stitches, hemorrhoids, and the fact that you just passed something the size of a watermelon from your body. Movement is not easy right now! So think sweet and simple: For the first few days, walk your baby, slowly dance with your baby in your arms, or sway back and forth with your baby in your arms. After one or two weeks (three or four if you had a Cesarean section), ask your doctor if you can start taking a walk daily.

Don't expect too much too soon. Take your time, and give your body some leeway. By going slowly the first couple of weeks, then increasing the amount you do daily, you will be ready to take on a healthy, more effective workout by the time your health-care specialist clears you.

▶ Note: Every Woman's Needs Are Unique

Because every birth and every woman's situation is different, follow your health-care professional's advice as to when to begin any exercise program after giving birth.

You're Never Too Old to Bounce Back

Hannah had wanted a baby ever since she could remember, but God had not given her one until she was considered too old to have one. Her husband, Elkanah, hearing the good news of her pregnancy, was as surprised and pleased as she was. Imagine becoming new parents at their ages! All their friends had been talking about retiring, and there they were, accumulating toys and baby clothes.

Samuel had been a little sweetheart from the minute she held him in her arms. Soon after his birth, Hannah had gingerly begun walking around the inside of the house just a little each day. One day, in a fit of joy she had held Samuel tightly in her arms and danced around the house with him. He seemed to love the idea, so she did it often—anything to keep moving so she could get back into shape.

Knowing she had to take it easy for the first couple of months, gradually she added deep knee bends, then walking to the market, carrying Samuel in a little basket Elkanah had made. It wasn't long before Hannah began to see a difference in the way she looked and felt. Her body was getting back into shape; her baby was healthy and thriving; and she and Elkanah had never been happier. Smiling to herself, she wondered, *Who says I'm too old to be a mother?*

—Scripture reference: 1 Samuel 1

▲ ▲ ▲

8 | Encouragement for Those with Postpartum Depression

Many women experience some sort of depression after having a baby. "Baby blues" are normal, typically mild, and in most cases, they will go away on their own.

For some women, baby blues are more severe and turn into *postpartum depression*. I'll show you how to tell the difference.

How Do I Know If I Have the Baby Blues?

Symptoms begin within one to three days after delivery and can last a few weeks. These include:

- crying spells
- depression
- anxiety
- mood swings
- irritability
- restlessness
- anger
- excessive worry
- forgetfulness
- insomnia
- feelings of inadequacy

- feelings of failure
- feelings of resentfulness

How Do I Know If I Have Postpartum Depression?

Symptoms begin within the first four weeks and can last several months. These include:

- all of the same symptoms for baby blues
- panic attacks
- loss of self-esteem
- feelings of guilt
- feelings of inadequacy and worthlessness
- impaired memory and confusion
- a sense of hopelessness and despair
- inability to care for yourself or your baby
- negative feelings toward your baby and/or spouse

Many factors physiologically and psychologically contribute to baby blues and postpartum depression. As I said, for most of you, the baby blues will be mild and will disappear in a short time. For those of you who experience postpartum depression, hang in there. It, too, will go away in time. If, however, at any time you feel that you are not getting better or might be a danger to yourself or your child, call your health-care provider immediately.

As I stated previously, Nicole didn't sleep through the night for the first seven months, but during my first week with her I was breast-feeding every two hours. I hadn't slept. I was exhausted, and looking back, most likely experiencing some baby blues.

One evening, after my being awake for days, Nicole would not settle down. She cried continuously no matter what I did. I rocked her for hours and tried feeding and changing her. Enduring this stressful situation in the middle of the night, all alone for four hours straight, I finally had had it. I couldn't deal with it anymore. All of my patience, strength, and normally loving thoughts disappeared, and I just wanted to toss my baby across the room to make her stop. With tears streaming down my face, I carried Nicole to Ben and asked him for help. All I asked for was one hour—one hour of sleep so that I could deal with her once again in a loving manner. Exhaustion and the baby blues had taken their toll on me. Thankfully, as the days went on, things did get better, and even though I continued to get very little sleep, I was better able to handle it. I am fortunate that my husband was there to help me during this critical time. If you are a single mother, you may want to keep a list of friends, family members, and neighbors who would be more than glad to help you out in times like these.

Baby blues can feel as if they are getting the best of you, and they may for a short period of time. But that's the key: typically they won't last. In order to lessen their effect, try exercising. The chemicals that your body naturally produces during exercise will be one of the biggest factors in turning around postpartum depression. You should also avoid caffeine, alcohol, and foods with additives and preservatives. If after this, however, you still do not find relief from your depression, seek help immediately from your health-care provider.

A Case in Point

Angie was so excited about her first pregnancy. She experienced a relatively easy delivery and couldn't wait to get home with her newborn. Yet twenty-four hours after her baby was born, something changed in her, and she felt as if she had no control over her nerves and emotions. It all started with a strong sense of anxiety if she wasn't holding her son; therefore, she began holding him nonstop, even while he slept. Whenever her husband tried to take him for a moment to give her a break, she screamed and started crying. In fact, she cried most of the day for no reason at all.

Not knowing what to do or how to help, her husband called Angie's mother. Her mother tried to get Angie to rest and sleep while she cared for the baby, but Angie refused to let him go. Her mother tried to take the baby out for a walk so Angie could rest, but Angie grew so nervous about being separated from her son that she grew hysterical.

Tension surged, and her mother suggested seeking the help of a doctor for medication. Angie didn't want to stop breast-feeding in order to take medication and became so angry that she threw her mother and her packed bag out the door—even though they had always been extremely close. Angie couldn't understand what was happening or why she was acting that way.

Angie's husband decided he had to take drastic action. He began by taking over nighttime feedings, using milk Angie pumped during the day. And he didn't allow her to hold the baby between 9 PM and 6 AM. He locked himself and the baby in another room even though she pounded on the door and wept.

After days of this, Angie realized that no matter how much she cried he wouldn't unlock the door—and she started resting. The more rest she got, the better she became. After a couple of weeks they were able to share the responsibility of nighttime care and day-time care when he was home from work. The anxiety lessened, but Angie still cried at the drop of a hat. It wasn't until six weeks after the delivery that Angie began to feel like her old self. The anxiety was gone, and the crying jags became infrequent.

It was a long and difficult six weeks, and looking back she realized the cause was postpartum depression. She made note, however, that when she experienced postpartum depression, she didn't recognize it while she was going through it. Therefore, it is important for the people around you to take control over the situation and seek help for you if needed.

PART III | Fueling for Bouncing Back

9 | Food by God: The Un-Diet

Have you noticed that social life in this country centers around food? We never arrange to meet a friend just to talk—we always meet for coffee. And it's hardly ever just coffee; it's coffee *and* . . . Since Eve offered Adam a taste of that piece of fruit, women have been focused on food as a way of bringing people together. And why not? It works! Even Jesus fed the five thousand before He delivered the Sermon on the Mount. There's nothing wrong with enjoying a meal or a healthy snack and beverage with friends and family. What's often wrong is the *type* of food we put into our mouths, and *how often* we put it there.

What, when, and how much you eat, and whether you exercise or not, are typically a result of your upbringing. Your current habits and routines are a product of learned behavior, or a response to your lifestyle. As a result, some of us exercise and some don't. Some of us eat too much and some too little. Some of us eat when we're happy, and some when we're sad.

The one thing we all have in common, however, is that these habits have taken us a lifetime to develop. Unfortunately for most of us, we have perfected poor and unhealthy habits that God did not intend for our bodies. The good news is that for many women, pregnancy forces them to think more carefully about what they're eating and provides an opportunity to seek out a healthier path.

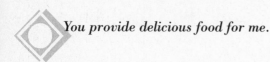

You provide delicious food for me.

—Psalm 23:5 TLB

Since you have chosen to read this book, you are probably asking yourself some critical questions, such as: *Are the habits I currently have regarding nutrition and exercise the ones I want to cultivate and keep? Are these habits the healthiest for my body? Are these habits the healthiest for my baby, and the ones I want to instill in my children? Or is there a better, healthier way?*

Looking at me, you would see someone who is petite, thin, and loves to exercise. You might question what I could possibly know about your situation or how difficult it could be for you to lose weight, develop healthy habits, or bounce back after a pregnancy. I'm not about to stand in a pulpit and preach to anyone because I realize we all have our own issues and past conditioning. Nor am I going to say that changing your habits is going to be a snap. But if you truly desire to change, the change *will* come once you replace your old habits with new, life-giving ones.

How do I know this? Because like you, I'm a real person who has had issues with food, and I have had to recognize and change my own nutritional and exercise habits. I had to get to the point where I *wanted* to take care of my body. Without my desire to change, it never would have happened.

I have friends who describe themselves as "exercise-intolerant," and others whose eating habits are not conducive to a healthy lifestyle. Whatever holds *you* back from being all you are capable of may be different for every other person who reads this book. What isn't different, however, is how it is addressed. All of us need to face our own personal situations, want to change for the better, and then work toward replacing old habits with new ones.

My Battle with Food

I began participating in gymnastics when I was a small child. By second grade, my mother and coaches felt that I should be placed on a team whose goal was to train and produce Olympic athletes. I was required to take gymnastic classes three times a week for three to four hours at a time. By fourth grade, my gym time had increased to six days a week for five hours a day.

From the age of six I had been weighed daily. At that time I was the smallest member on the team, and I weighed forty-nine pounds. I will never forget the day when I was told that I *had* to weigh forty-eight pounds and I needed to lose weight. From that point on, I endured a regimented weight control and literally watched the scales morning and night.

When I reached seventh grade, something in me changed. Like most girls that age, I became very interested in friends at school, causing me to be less interested in gymnastics. Even though I had loved gymnastics up to that point, I thought I would love hanging out with my friends even more. My mother and I argued daily over whether I went to the gym and worked out. I looked for every excuse not to go. We used to carpool with other gymnasts, and when they arrived to pick me up, I hid. Finally the coaches told my mother that I didn't want to be there, that I wasn't progressing, and that I should no longer be on the team. My mother was devastated, but I was elated.

I soon became involved with a group of girls who weren't the best influence on me. It seemed all we did was get into trouble, and eventually they weren't so fun to hang around with because of this. The only way I knew how to break away from them was to go back to the gym because it would leave me with no free time. By then, however, almost a year had passed and my body had changed considerably. Puberty had set in, and I had grown four inches and added twenty pounds. Physically, I was a completely different person from who I was before. When I rejoined the Olympic training team, I had gone from being the smallest gymnast to the largest.

As soon as I went back to the team, weight control immediately became the order of the day. If I weighed more than one hundred pounds, I was kicked out of the gym, which happened weekly. If I was even close to being over my weight goal, my coaches didn't speak to me during practices. They didn't correct or encourage me. They only gave me an evil glare, as if I were despicable. My best friend in gymnastics was very short and stocky, which at that time was not okay for a gymnast. Our coaches made her wear a sign on her back that said *PIG*. For years that one incident bothered me, and I now realize what repercussions it had on me as a young girl.

For fear that I would have to wear that sign, and to avoid the humiliation I was enduring daily in the gym, I *had* to take control of my weight. I learned how to manipulate the scale by sliding the weight slightly to the left of the notch, and I learned how to manipulate my eating habits to get the results I wanted.

At that point, what I ate (or *didn't* eat) became an obsession for me. It got so bad that I could no longer eat in front of anyone. Instead I woke up at 2 AM and snuck to the kitchen to get something to eat so that no one would see me eat it. But due to puberty and the weight most young teenagers add, this wasn't working well for me in the gym. I tried diet pills for a short time, but eventually I found that not eating worked better. If I did eat, I purged afterward. I mastered not eating at all.

I stayed on the team for another year but could no longer endure the anxiety I felt, so I quit. By then I was a sophomore and joined the high-school gymnastics team instead. That was fun, and for the first time in my life, I felt no pressure about my weight. As a result, my weight increased considerably until I was the heaviest I had ever been. It wasn't long afterward that my old habits of manipulating food started taking over my life once again. By eleventh grade I was the thinnest I had ever been. It never occurred to me that those habits could have an adverse affect on my health, so I continued them right through college.

I can't think of many college students with great eating habits, but mine were the worst. If I didn't eat at all, I was really happy. One day I saw a program on television on anorexia and bulimia. Instead of scaring me, it made me want to act and look that way. I had no idea what I was doing to my body and no concept that I was harming it. That was simply my routine, my eating habits, what I knew. No one said, "This is the healthy way, and this is the unhealthy way, to take care of your body."

I went through my college years and chiropractic school not eating and not exercising. It wasn't until I began work as a chiropractor that I realized my lifestyle wasn't working for me. Because I wasn't eating, I wasn't thinking properly. My mind was always in a fog because I was so tired all the time. I could never give 100 percent to my job simply because I didn't have the strength, stamina, or clarity of mind to do it. Often when I adjusted my patients, I almost passed out when straightening back up. I had to grab the wall to steady myself regularly. My back, as well as all my joints, hurt all the time. My body was breaking down because I wasn't taking care of it properly. I realized there was a problem and knew I couldn't move to the next level in my life unless things changed.

Even though I had been a Christian since the age of five, I hadn't attended church for several years. I was tired of my life and wanted a peace and calm in it that I wasn't experiencing. I decided to recommit my time to God. Once I did, God showed me a better path.

A short time later God brought my future husband, Ben, into my life. We met at a chiropractic seminar and began dating long-distance, since I lived in Pennsylvania and he lived in Florida. I learned what he did, how he lived his life, and his desire to help and serve others. He was such a positive example that he motivated and inspired me to try to turn my life around. I saw that God could really use Ben for His purpose more than He could use me simply because of my frail and unhealthy body. I realized that without a lot of changes in my life, I would limit my usefulness to God.

For the first time I realized that what I was doing to my body was unhealthy and my lifestyle was only a temporary fix. Along with opening my own chiropractic office came the desire to live a healthier life. I needed a way of eating that would last a lifetime. I focused on the changes I wanted to make. The problems for me *then* were twofold: One, I had a distorted image of what I should look like and how much I should weigh. It wasn't okay to be overweight, so I had to find a healthy way to deal with that. The second problem was that I had developed habits, and habits are addictive, just as smoking or drugs may be. It would be difficult to break them or change them. I knew that I faced a struggle, but I wanted to find a healthier approach to eating and exercise.

As Ben and I became closer, he began teaching me the concepts that are now in this book. He taught me how to take care of my body—my Body by God. Making the changes necessary, however, didn't happen overnight. It was a *process*. I had to learn to focus on healthy eating habits instead of *not*-eating habits. For you it might be the reverse. Either way, it's all about desire, motivation, and trust.

First, you must have a deep *desire* to break old, unhealthy habits and replace them with new, life-giving ones. Second, you must have the *motivation* to change, and third, and most important of all, you must *trust*. If you trust God to help you change, He will give you the strength you need to change your lifestyle.

Your One Body

Haven't you yet learned that your body is the home of the Holy Spirit God gave you, and that he lives within you? Your own body does not belong to you. For God has bought you with a great price. So use

every part of your body to give glory back to God,
because he owns it.

—1 Corinthians 6:19–20 TLB

God has given you only one body. Your assignment is to take care of it. Start slowly, integrate Food by God into your daily diet, and you'll soon see a difference in how you feel. Just remember that no one is perfect all of the time. You will have days when you do not do as well at eating Food by God. Don't beat yourself up when that happens. Just do better the next time. The important thing is to begin improving your health now, one step at a time. It won't take long for you to notice that you have more energy, a more fit body, and a more hopeful outlook on life. You'll have more strength and you'll live longer, which means you can do more to help people and fulfill God's purpose for your life. Food by God and the Un-Diet really do work!

▶ Note: Further Help with Eating Disorders

For some of you, this may not be enough. Years of eating disorders might require more help than any book can give you. If this is your case, seek the help of specialists who deal with eating disorders.

I always think that pregnant women aren't counting correctly when they say they are eating for two. Actually when you're pregnant, you are eating for dozens: yourself, your unborn child, God, and all the people God will use you to bless if you live longer by eating healthier, and all the people God will bless through your healthy child's life as well. Awesome responsibility, right? If that doesn't make you want to put the right things into your mouth, I don't know what will!

Some of you have families who won't support this change in eating habits. If this is the case, try to slowly introduce one good Food by God at a time to each meal. Give your family options. It may mean that you have to cook a few additional items initially, but hopefully you will be able to integrate some of the Food by God into your family's diet.

The Un-Diet

The Un-Diet is the way God intended people to eat. It's also the answer to America's obesity crisis, as well as many other health problems. If you want to eat your fill and still look and feel great, the Un-Diet is for you!

Designed by my husband, Dr. Ben Lerner, this plan for eating well for maximum health contains foods that are neither bad-tasting nor expensive. It's often possible to buy foods such as fruits and vegetables, rice and potatoes in bulk for less money than you'd think, especially when compared to eating meals out or buying prepared foods. Protein-rich foods such as fish and poultry are very affordable as well. There are so many health food stores around the country now that it's also easy to find organic foods that are chemical-free. (Sometimes organic food is a little more expensive, but the flavor is wonderful, and it is so much better for you that it's worth the extra cost.)

> *The Israelites were puzzled when they saw it. "What is it?" they asked. And Moses told them, "It is the food the LORD has given you."*
>
> —Exodus 16:15

Food preparation is also less of a chore when you prepare several meals at once. You can cook many foods in volume and provide meals for several days. For traveling or when you spend the day at work, packing food in containers or resealable plastic bags makes instant picnics easy and fun, whether your entire family is together or you are alone. Wherever you are, you can make eating Food by God an easy part of your life. The Un-Diet Food Guide on pages

104-121 discusses when to eat which types of food for maximum benefit and good balance.

Myths the Un-Diet Dissolves

Following are some popular myths about dieting countered by Un-Diet truths:

Diet Myth #1: Diet = Deprivation.
Un-Diet Truth: The Un-Diet is not about eating only bland, tasteless foods, restricting portions, or cutting calories. In fact, while the Un-Diet does recommend certain foods, if you follow the Un-Diet Food Guide found on pages 104-121, you do not have to change the foods you eat at all.

Diet Myth #2: Eat like an elephant, look like an elephant.
Un-Diet Truth: If you are eating the foods in the way God intended you to (following the Un-Diet Food Guide), you can eat all you want and you will *never* look like an elephant.

Diet Myth #3: If you crave, you cave (once you cheat or go off your diet, it's over).
Un-Diet Truth: Taking short vacations from proper eating is part of the Un-Diet. Eating a food you crave is actually part of the plan.

Diet Myth #4: You can trick the body into thinness and better health.
Un-Diet Truth: God's body cannot be tricked; we should look on it in awe. Diets that restrict foods or use only one kind of food category, such as a protein-only diet, may trick the body into change in the short term.

However, they never work in the long term. Eliminating an entire food group cannot be healthy because God would not have placed those foods on the earth in the first place if He had not intended that we eat them.

The Un-Diet uses a balance of foods *including* fruits, vegetables, whole grains such as oats and basmati rice, as well as protein, all eaten at the right time to create real, lasting health and thinness.

Diet Myth #5: It's best to get a balance of protein, fats, and carbohydrates at every meal.

Un-Diet Truth: Your body needs varying amounts of carbohydrates, proteins, and fats at different *times* throughout the day. Also, the Body by God does not digest protein and carbohydrates the same way, so they should not be consumed in large amounts together.

Diet Myth #6: There is a cookie-cutter diet that works for all people or all people with certain backgrounds or body types.

Un-Diet Truth: God made people like snowflakes; no two are exactly alike.

Diet Myth #7: *Low-, reduced-, -free, no-* foods are *health and diet foods*, and food that is good for you is expensive.

Un-Diet Truth: Synthetic, refined, or chemically altered foods that say *low-fat, reduced-cholesterol, lactose-free, no-sugar*, etc., will never grant long-term health or thinness. Anything man creates for the Body by God to eat cannot be considered health and diet food. Additionally, these foods are expensive. Food by God is the only health and diet food there is, and overall it costs a lot less.

Food by God

God created specific foods for your body to utilize in order to produce maximum health. These are what we call Food by God, and He has endowed them with the perfect amounts of nutrients in perfect balance for the body to use. It all works together, in the Body by God, to produce Health by God.

The job of the digestive system is to process and absorb the nutrients in the food you eat. Every cell, every organ, every type of fluid in your Body by God is designed to fulfill a specific role in this process. It's incredible when you think about it. What's even more amazing to me is that while I was pregnant, all these organs and systems were being formed in my baby as she grew in my womb.

> *You made all the delicate, inner parts of my body, and knit them together in my mother's womb. Thank you for making me so wonderfully complex! It is amazing to think about. Your workmanship is marvelous—and how well I know it. You were there while I was being formed in utter seclusion!*
> —Psalm 139:13–15 TLB

Food by God is the best source of optimum health, for both you and your baby, both while you are pregnant *and* after the baby is born. Food by God is crammed with the digestive enzymes, vitamins, minerals, and countless other goodies every human being needs to live life to the fullest in his or her Body by God. It wouldn't be wise to ignore it!

▶ Tip: Food by God Is Smart Food!

Food by God and all the vitamins, minerals, and other elements it contains are put together by the intelligence of God. Food by God is smart food. When you eat Food by God, such as an apple or a carrot, it knows what to do inside the Body by God, and the intelligent Body by God knows what to do with it.

Food by God List
The following is a selection of the most beneficial Food by God:

Fruits

- Apples
- Bananas
- Blackberries
- Blueberries
- Cantaloupe
- Currants
- Grapefruit
- Grapes
- Honeydew melons
- Kiwi
- Lemons
- Limes
- Mangoes
- Nectarines
- Oranges
- Peaches
- Pears
- Pineapple
- Plums
- Prunes
- Raisins
- Raspberries
- Strawberries
- Tangerines
- Watermelon

Good Carbohydrates

- All-natural, whole grain, chemical-free, sugar-free breads, flours, and cereals
- Barley
- Brown, jasmine, and basmati rice
- Buckwheat
- Cream of brown rice
- Grits
- Millet
- Oats
- Other hot whole grain cereals (barley, quinoa, rye, spelt, millet, flax)
- Rice cakes, rice noodles, puffed rice cereal
- Rye
- Spelt
- Unprocessed soy

Starchy Vegetables

- Corn
- Peas
- Potatoes
- Squash
- Sweet potatoes

Vegetables

- Alfalfa
- Artichokes
- Arugula
- Asparagus
- Bamboo shoots
- Beets
- Broccoli
- Brussels sprouts
- Cabbage
- Carrots
- Cauliflower
- Celery
- Collard greens
- Cucumbers
- Eggplant
- Escarole
- Green beans
- Kale
- Lettuce: all kinds
- Mesclun
- Mustard greens
- Onions
- Parsley
- Parsnips
- Pea pods
- Portabello mushrooms
- Radishes
- Radicchio
- Scallions
- Seaweed
- Shallots
- Swiss chard
- Snap peas
- Spinach
- String beans
- Tomatoes (also considered fruit)
- Turnips
- Watercress
- Wheat grass
- Zucchini

Beans (Protein and Carbohydrate)

- Chickpeas
- Fresh soy
- Kidney
- Lentil
- Lima
- Navy
- Pinto
- White

Nuts (Fat and Protein)

- Almonds
- Brazil nuts
- Hazelnuts
- Pine nuts
- Walnuts

Seeds (Fat and Protein)

- Flax
- Pumpkin
- Sesame
- Sunflower

Good Proteins

Eggs

- Best are from organic, free-range chickens

Fish

- Grouper
- Halibut
- Mackerel
- Mahimahi
- Rainbow trout
- Salmon
- Sardines
- Sea bass
- Snapper
- Swordfish
- Trout
- Tuna
- Whitefish

Poultry

- Chicken/turkey breast (Best from organic free-range)

Red Meat

- From organic, grass-fed beef
- Lean beef

Good Fats

- Almonds/ almond butter
- Avocados
- Crushed flaxseed
- Extra-virgin coconut oil
- Fish oil
- Olives (oil: cold-pressed, extra-virgin)
- Tahini (sesame and olive oil)
- Organic fats in grass- and vegetable-fed beef, egg yolks, and chicken
- Walnuts

Beverages

- Almond, rice, or oat milk
- Herbal tea
- Fresh fruit and vegetable juices
- Water: reverse osmosis, distilled, fresh-spring, filtered

Condiments

(Condiments are not used in heavy amounts, so they can do little damage, unless they are from a chemical source.)

- All-natural hot sauce
- Basil, curry, dill, garlic, ginger, horseradish, mint, miso, mustard, paprika, parsley, rosemary, tarragon, and thyme
- Butter Buds (without hydrogenated oil)
- Ginger
- High-quality vinegar
- Lemon juice
- Natural mustards
- Sesame seeds
- Natural soy sauce or tamari
- Olive-oil-based and low-fat, chemical-free dressings
- Spices without MSG or hydrolyzed vegetable protein

Sweeteners

- Almond butter
- Brown rice syrup
- Fruit and fruit juice
- Honey
- Unrefined maple syrup
- Unsweetened, all-natural fruit jellies and syrups

Food by Man

This is food that man has either created or altered. On the flip side, it's food that God didn't intend your Body by God to eat on a regular basis. Food by Man is difficult, if not downright impossible, for your Body by God to digest and process. It hangs around inside your body and causes problems, such as hindering the processing of Food by God, creating pockets of excess fat, and breeding disease. Food by Man might taste good going down, but it usually makes you feel less than great both physically and emotionally.

Most Food by Man is made from dead components (all those things on the label you cannot pronounce), so it's logical that if there is nothing alive in it, it's not contributing much to *your* life. When you face a choice of eating Food by God that is alive and healthy (a perfectly ripe cantaloupe, for example), or Food by Man (a bag of chemicals, additives, and preservatives sprayed orange and deep-fried in artery-clogging saturated fat, for example), you need to remember that you are eating for dozens: the dozens of people God wants you to bless in your life. You need to be fully alive and well for Him to fully use you to be the blessing-dispenser He intends. I don't know about you, but I don't want to miss one single minute of God's plan for my life!

It's true that the Body by God is so wonderfully designed that it can process and utilize even bad fuel sources. But when you eat only Food by Man, and too much of it, even the Body by God gives up and cries for help. (It's called getting obese and/or sick.)

I've mentioned that some think that Food by God is more costly than Food by Man. But it isn't in the long run, because it costs much less than doctors' visits should you get sick. Seek out farmers' markets or small, fresh-produce grocery stores that buy from local farmers. Often costs are lower than at a typical larger grocery chain, and foods are fresher.

Warning: Food by Man may be hazardous to your health!

▶ Tip: Proper Fueling

If you fuel your body with Food by Man, the energy required to operate the digestive system becomes so great that power will be stolen from the other systems in the body. This is particularly dangerous because it will eventually weaken the Body by God immune system.

Fueling with Food by God will minimize the amount of power needed for digestion, leaving more energy for the rest of the body.

Don't you realize that all of you together are the house of God, and that the Spirit of God lives among you in his house? If anyone defiles and spoils God's home, God will destroy him. For God's home is holy and clean, and you are that home.

—1 Corinthians 3:16–17 TLB

With that caution from the Bible resounding in your head and heart, remind yourself every time you eat that Food by Man is toxic, and choose Food by God instead.

Here is a list of some foods that man has either made or tampered with, making them unbeneficial to your health:

- Pork
- Shellfish
- Sugar substitutes
- Hydrogenated oils
- Additives, colorings, flavorings, and preservatives
- Fast, refined, and fried foods
- Other animal products
- Dairy foods
- Caffeine
- Refined sugar
- Table salt
- White foods

Do Not Close the Book
After Reading This List!

It's true that reducing your use of these foods is part of the Un-Diet, but the real focus of the Un-Diet is on *adding* better choices from the Food by God list. If you work outside the home, or if you have children (and even a husband) who are used to eating lots of Food by Man, you may have trouble sticking to a Food by God lifestyle. The good news is that even the smallest shifts in diet *away* from Food by Man *toward* Food by God will produce noticeable improvements in the way you feel and in your overall health.

 One Mom's Story

Lisa had her hands full with three children under age twelve; the youngest was eight. And then she learned she was pregnant! She and her husband were surprised but happy. Unfortunately, Lisa was older and her eating habits had settled into a comfortable, though less healthy, routine. She had to start thinking about eating better for both herself and the baby.

Lisa's mother was delighted to be anticipating another grandchild, but instead of buying Lisa a baby book, she bought her a copy of *Body by God,* by Dr. Ben Lerner. She had been using some of the principles in the book, and she was not only looking great at sixty-two, she was feeling more like forty-seven. If she could change her eating habits and start exercising, so could Lisa.

Lisa loved the book and got excited about the concept of making little changes in her diet and lifestyle. She began adding one Food by God at each meal and walking for exercise. After several days of these two small adjustments in her life, she noticed that she really didn't want to eat a bag of potato chips in front of the television in the evening. She found herself fixing a plate of raw veggies instead. Her body was telling her what it wanted. Amazing!

By the end of her first trimester, Lisa was eating mostly from the Food by God List. (See pages 78-81.) She had incorporated several exercises into her daily routine, and she was feeling really good. Eventually Lisa delivered a healthy, eight-pound, three-ounce daughter with no complications.

Lisa chose to stay on the Body by God plan because she felt better when she was following it. She didn't force any part of it on her family, but gradually they, too, began to choose healthier snacks and meals. Little by little, the small changes Lisa made added up to one huge difference in her life and the lives of her family members.

▲ ▲ ▲

These small changes in diet especially help your new baby. He or she is not yet addicted to Food by Man, so you have a clean slate on which to write Food by God principles for that little boy or girl you just brought into the world.

Starting your baby out correctly is easy if you are breast-feeding. All you have to do is be sure *you* are eating Food by God so the nutrients pass to your baby through your milk. If you started eating Food by God while you were pregnant and have maintained those standards while bouncing back, you have already started your baby down the right nutrition path. If you didn't know about Food by God in time to do that, start now. Food by God and the Un-Diet are still the best plan for optimum health and energy. It's never too late to begin doing things right. When you look into that tiny, adorable face and realize what a responsibility you have to your child, how can you *not* make a shift in your food choices?

Teach a child to choose the right path, and when he is older he will remain upon it.
—**Proverbs 22:6** TLB

Next, let's discuss some of the foods I listed on page 83 as Food by Man, and why I included them.

God's D-List

If God is all-wise (and He is), then it makes sense for us to pay attention when He says not to do something. In Leviticus 11 God listed animals that He considered not good for people to eat: pigs, camels, dogs, and horses all made God's D-list (D for *delete*). If you eat them, you will neither die nor be kept out of heaven for doing so, but there are other reasons for not eating them. Consider the pig: high in saturated fat and cholesterol, its by-products (ham, sausage, and bacon) are full of salt, sugar, and various chemicals, making them harmful to the Body by God's digestive system.

And then there are shellfish: lobsters, crabs, clams, and shrimp, to name a few. In Leviticus 11:12, the Bible forbids eating anything living in the water that does not have fins and scales. The main diet of shellfish is fish droppings, and with all the toxins and pollution in the water . . . well, you can figure it out.

Here are some other Foods by Man on God's D-List:

Sugar Substitutes

Sugar itself lowers your energy, can produce mood swings, causes your teeth to rot, and can make you gain weight, but there's hardly a human alive that doesn't love the sweet stuff. So man invented sugar substitutes: chemical concoctions as an alternative to sugar. If you don't think they're dangerous, consider the fact that when a sugar substitute is added to a food, *by law* the manufacturer must put a warning label on the package. Sugar, salt, and fat substitutes are dangerous to the Body by God.

Hydrogenated Oils, Additives, Colorings, Flavorings, and Preservatives

Hydrogenated oils (even partially hydrogenated oils) contain trans-fatty acids and are artificially processed vegetable oils. Pumping hydrogen into them retards spoilage and prevents melting at room temperature. These are found in margarine, fast foods, prepared foods, and baked goods. If it's a quick snack food, it probably has hydrogenated oils in it, and you should definitely avoid it.

And then there are the additives, colorings, flavorings, and preservatives—pure chemicals foreign to your Body by God. Fast, refined, and fried foods contain many of these problem compounds and should be avoided, because they supply no nutritive value and block your colon, making you feel fatigued and groggy. They literally drain your Body by God of its power, cause fat deposits in the most unwanted places, and promote several serious diseases, including colon cancer. Why eat anything that does all that harm?

Animal Products

Animals raised naturally (free-range), eating grass and vegetables, are healthier by far than those raised in commercial enterprises to supply the large grocery stores.

Dairy

Cow's milk was designed for baby cows; God never intended it for human consumption. And, of course, any antibiotics, steroids, hormones, and other drugs that are injected into the cows to speed production do end up in the milk, and therefore, in your cereal bowl. Any products made from cow's milk have the same problem. If you are worried about calcium for your Body by God, you'll find the best source in green, leafy vegetables. (That's where the cows get it from, by the way.) Good substitutes for cow's milk are almond milk and rice milk, available at health food stores and many grocery stores as well.

Caffeine

Caffeine is a stimulant that affects your heart functions, alters the flow of blood in your veins, and overstimulates your digestive system and glands. It seems to manipulate the body's level of energy, but in reality, it causes your energy level to crash eventually, which requires more caffeine to get it back up again, so it can crash again . . . and on the cycle goes.

Refined Sugar

The sugarcane plant is the only natural form of sugar there is. What you find in your sugar bowl is refined from the sugarcane plant and has basically become a concentrated chemical with no nutritive value. Refined sugar actually alters the physiology of the brain. Extended use can be linked to many diseases, including obesity, because excess sugar ends up being stored as fat. It's entirely possible to become addicted to sugar. My advice is to break the habit now. No one is born with a sweet tooth; it's acquired.

Table Salt

Read a few labels, and you'll be surprised to see salt as one of the ingredients. Why does applesauce need salt? Beats me. But there it is on the label. Americans have not only a sweet tooth for refined sugar, they have an acidic tooth for salt. Salt puts so much stress on the Body by God that you should avoid it totally.

White Foods

These are foods made from white flour—flour that has been bleached or bromated to make it nicer in appearance and finer in quality, not as coarse and chewy as whole grain flours. Breads, pastas, and pastries made from white flour have almost no nutrition left in them. They fill you up *and* fill you out, without providing any nutrients.

Faced with all these poor choices that are so prevalent in our American lifestyle, what's a person supposed to do? Eat Food by God. Fruits and vegetables are truly Food by God and good choices for your Body by God. They are absorbed well and quickly by the body, fill you up, provide healthy and high-quality nutrition, are easy to grow or buy, and cost very little. These should make up the bulk of your diet. Their high fiber helps with the processing of nutrients and the elimination of the bulk not needed by your Body by God.

10 | Understanding the Different Types of Fuels

Food comes in three types: carbohydrates, proteins, and fats. All Food by God fits within these categories. To be healthy, you need nutrients from all three categories, in the correct balance. Medical science doesn't fully understand how it all works together, even after several thousands of years of studying the human body. That's because God is so much bigger and wiser than we are, and He knew exactly what He was doing when He created the first human body. What we *do* know, however, is enough to keep us all busy for the rest of our lives studying His principles and applying them to our lives.

Carbohydrates

No engine runs without power, not even the human engine. Power comes from eating carbohydrates. Natural, untampered-with Food by God containing carbohydrates slowly converts to sugar (not the same white granules sold on the supermarket shelves). We're talking about blood sugar here, which provides a sustained level of power.

Blood sugar is interesting. I had a friend who nearly died behind the wheel of her car because of low blood sugar. Ellie had a job that involved traveling around the country and visiting in the homes of many people. Everywhere she went, her hostesses offered her coffee *and* a baked good—full of white flour, refined sugar, and real butter or some other fat. It's interesting to note that in her entire five years of doing that job, not once did anyone offer her a healthy treat, such as fruit! Not wanting to be impolite, Ellie always accepted whatever they offered and dutifully ate it. She was, after all, trying to make a good impression on those women so they would get involved in the project she was promoting.

After about six months, Ellie began to feel less well than usual. She chalked it up to not getting enough sleep and had more coffee and baked goods . . . to keep her going. Gradually Ellie learned this hard fact of life: refined carbohydrates generate an appetite for even more refined carbohydrates. If she didn't have a certain amount of sweets, she felt extremely tired, and her mind could not seem to get out of first gear. She also noticed that about twenty minutes after she ate a donut or pastry, she had her usual bubbly energy level back. The trouble was it didn't last. In about three hours she needed another refined carbohydrate fix.

Her blood sugar was riding a seesaw: soaring, crashing, soaring, and crashing. She was addicted to sugar and didn't know it. This went on for three years.

One day when Ellie was driving through the mountains of Colorado on a back country road, she suddenly found her car sitting sideways on the road, with the nose pointed downward at the very edge of a sheer drop into a heavily treed valley more than five hundred feet deep. There was no guardrail. She remembered pushing the brake pedal, but not very hard, as if she were operating in a fog. Suddenly she felt as if someone else's foot was on top of hers, grinding her foot into the pedal and bringing the car to a stop. There was no one else in the car.

Looking down the precipice below her, she shook her head to clear it. Her immediate reaction was fear of what had almost happened, and then she realized that God had protected her from a horrible accident, or even death. All for a few donuts that developed into a deadly eating habit! Once her heart stopped racing, she realized that something was terribly wrong with her reaction time.

And second, she realized she needed to pay attention to what she had been eating.

A few days later, at her next stopover, she visited with a woman who was a nutritionist. Ellie was not feeling great, and her hostess picked up on it, asking what was wrong. Ellie told her story, and thankfully she had a listener who knew something about prevention through good nutrition. Bottom line: Ellie stopped eating sweets and donuts and started eating Food by God—although it wasn't called that back in the seventies because my husband hadn't written his book yet! My friend Ellie still has an occasional donut or pastry when she craves one, but the state of her health is near perfect. Her story is a great example of how truly devastating Food by Man can be.

God designed carbohydrates to be broken down gradually and converted to blood glucose (sugar) in order to provide a sustained level of power that is safe and effective. Carbohydrate-derived power burns fat inside the body, holds water inside the body's tissues, and keeps the body from burning its own muscles in order to produce energy.

Fruits and Vegetables

If you're looking for nearly perfect food and a source for carbohydrates, look no further than fruits and vegetables. You don't have to do anything to them except wash them. They have high water content that is loaded with vitamins, minerals, antioxidants, and enzymes—all of the highest quality, occurring naturally (not synthetically produced by man). The Body by God is also mostly water, so fruits and vegetables are easily absorbed and efficiently utilized. Their high-fiber content also moves the unnecessary bulk through your digestive tract and out of your body. And the taste of just-picked corn on the cob or peaches ripened in the sun and just plucked from the tree simply cannot be explained in words! If you've experienced those incredible flavors, you know what I mean. (If you *haven't* experienced them, put this book down and go find a farm stand with fresh produce!)

Apple vs. Broccoli

Fruits	Vegetables
Increase blood sugar	Little blood sugar effect
Many carbohydrates	Few carbohydrates
Potentially yeast-forming	Non-yeast-forming and potentially yeast-fighting

Because fruit contains a significant amount of carbohydrates and sugar, it is best eaten only in the morning and does not combine well with other foods. Vegetables, on the other hand, are great to eat anytime or with almost anything.

Follow the Body by God Un-Diet directions to make the best use of the two top Foods by God in the carbohydrate category.

Starchy Vegetables

Potatoes, sweet potatoes, yams, squash, corn, and peas are also nearly perfect. Unlike fruit, these vegetables must be cooked.

Beans

And in addition to being classified as carbohydrates, fresh beans are also clean proteins. (See the Un-Diet guidelines on page 114 for proper use of fresh beans.)

Whole Grains

Brown, basmati, and jasmine rice, oats, rye, and barley are excellent sources of carbohydrates, containing readily usable and high-quality nutrients for your Body by God. When cooking these grains, allow twenty minutes to one hour (depending on the grain). A good rule of thumb is that the more whole a grain is, the longer it will take to cook. Whole grains contain the shell and all the original nutrients and fiber.

The Whole Grain Rule: Farmed, Not Refined

The Whole Grain Rule states: the less refined and the more whole (the closer to the farm) the grain is, the more properly it is processed inside the body and the more nutrients it still contains.

Whole Grain Breads, Cereals, and Pastas

These are the best offerings from the Food by Man category because they are closest to the natural state. They are partially refined, however, so they don't break down in the Body by God as well as unrefined whole grains. The less refined and the less tampered with they are, the better for your Body by God.

Refined Grains, Cereals, Pastas (White Foods)

These are refined beyond use. They contain no nutrients, and the Body by God cannot process them. Avoid these chemically treated and tampered-with products, as they cause many problems inside the body.

▶ Tip: The Use of Grains in Your Feed Bag

Whole, close-to-the-farm grains are mostly healthy. You should limit them, however, according to the Un-Diet plan due to the blood sugar and acid-causing effects that they have on the Body by God.

Gluten found in wheat and wheat products is a common cause of food sensitivity reactions in the Body by God. These reactions cause things such as yeast infections, inflammatory bowel conditions, skin problems, and reflux. Therefore, they may need to be drastically reduced or eliminated in some Un-Diets.

Sugar (Any Anything with Sugar in It)

Sugar comes in several varieties: white, brown, high-fructose corn syrup, cane, raw, honey, and fruit. The refined sugars are white, brown, and high-fructose corn syrup. Less-refined sugars (cane and raw, for example) still give a high dose of concentrated sugar and are still unhealthy, although the body can process those types a bit more easily than the refined types of sugar. Because honey and the sugar in fruit have not been tampered with, they are the easiest forms of sugar for the Body by God to process.

Watch Out for Too Many Carbohydrates!

Eating too many carbohydrates can be hazardous to your health. The high levels of blood sugar this produces can cause pancreatic, glandular, brain, and blood problems. The extra stress put on your Body by God can produce other health problems as well. On top of that, your body will store the unused sugar as fat. High blood pressure, high cholesterol levels, and arterial problems can also result when you consistently consume too many carbohydrates. All of this is too high a price to pay for a few moments of gastronomic pleasure.

The Body by God needs carbohydrates to produce power, but the amount it needs is relative to how much energy you expend. It's easy to see how an imbalance between input and output can cause health problems.

Often in life timing is everything, even *when* you eat *what*. You should consume the foods that provide your Body by God with power (the carbohydrates) in the morning, when you're gathering your strength for the day ahead. Another optimum time to eat carbohydrates is before or right after hard exercise.

On the flip side, you don't need a large dose of power-fuel just before you go to bed or for periods of little activity. This is just the opposite of typical American dietary habits, where many eat large volumes of carbohydrates just before bedtime as a sort of reward for making it through the day. This makes your body spend the entire night digesting the carbohydrate load and leaves you feeling tired in the morning, even though you have supposedly been resting all night. In reality, you've been sleeping, but your body has been hard at work for six to eight hours!

Proteins

In many ways, proteins are the opposite of carbohydrates. There is protein in all foods, but the most abundant source is animal products, particularly the flesh. Animal products, however, are not a good source of energy-producing power. (Animal products *are* a good source of those all-important building blocks of health and energy: amino acids, which build and repair the body tissues.) Animal proteins do not cause blood sugar to increase.

Nuts, Seeds, Beans, Whole Grains, and Vegetables

These foods contain fewer proteins and amino acids, but they do have some, and the fact that they also provide carbohydrates and other nutrients is a plus. *Combining* Food by God from this category with food from other categories can provide an amino-acid-rich concentrated protein. A word of caution: high-protein diets can be toxic and hard to digest. If you consume too many animal products on a regular basis, you've stepped over the line from Food by God into Food by Man.

Proteins and Carbohydrates Don't Digest Well Together

Different types of food require different digestion processes, so eating large quantities of both carbohydrates and proteins together gives the Body by God a difficult task, causing improper or incomplete absorption of the nutrients from both categories of food. Instead, your meals should focus on either carbohydrates or on proteins or be a digestible balance of both. Think of it as stuffing stringy celery stalks and onion peelings down the garbage disposal in your sink and then turning it on. (If you've made the mistake of putting either of these things in the disposal before, you can already anticipate what will happen!) The celery strings will wrap themselves around the teeth of the disposal until it stops working, and the onion peelings will simply coat the whole mess with slime and keep it from operating as it should. There's nothing wrong with either the celery sticks or the onion peelings, but together, they totally clog up the garbage disposal.

Do not combine: eggs and fruit, fruit and vegetables, meat and potatoes, spaghetti and meatballs, eggs and toast and hash browns, pepperoni and pizza, bread and meat, and so on. All these combinations provide too many carbohydrates with too many proteins at once and cause disastrous collisions inside the fuel processing system.

Fats

When it comes to the Body by God's ability to handle fats, there are good fats, okay fats, and really bad fats.

Fats derived from animal products, nuts, seeds, and vegetables contain necessary nutrients for the health of your brain, glands, and cells. Fats insulate and protect the Body by God, helping it move and absorb minerals. Eating fats makes you feel more satisfied than when you eat other foods. Food absorption also slows down when you eat fats, so your body maintains better control of blood sugar.

Good Fats

Good fats such as *omega-3 fatty acids* benefit the Body by God, especially the cardiovascular system, the joints, and the immune system. Omega-3 fatty acids occur naturally in fish, fish oils, animals that have been grass- and vegetable-fed and raised naturally, flaxseed, and walnuts. Salmon, sardines, mackerel, halibut, cod, and tuna are excellent sources of omega-3.

Almonds and evening primrose oil are not omega-3 fats, but they are helpful in balancing acidic diets and in regulating hormone production. Extra-virgin olive oil, coconut oil, and avocados are also sources of good fats that are not omega-3.

Fats to Avoid

Fats to avoid because they are damaging to your Body by God are other omega fats prevalent in processed foods, commercial meats, and nut, seed, and vegetable oils. (Notice the missing 3; we're not talking about omega-3 fats now, just omega fats.)

Saturated fats are found in palm and coconut oils, and in animals raised commercially as a food source. It's true that saturated fats do have some benefits, but too many of them in a diet are harmful. (Note that coconut oil contains several helpful properties and is a good, stable source of cooking oil.)

Because they are very unstable and break down into compounds that are unhealthy for the Body by God (especially when they are heated), vegetable, nut, bean, and seed oils are to be avoided.

The worst fats are *trans fats*, which contain hydrogenated (or partially hydrogenated) oils. (See the Food by Man listed on page 83.) These oils have been altered by man, and the body can no longer utilize them. The body cannot even break them down. They are basically unprocessed fats that the body has to store someplace—usually in either a dangerous or very visible place.

Bad Fats

- Fats found in fried, greasy, fast foods
- Hydrogenated oils (trans fats)
- Milk fat/cream
- Nongrass-, nonorganic-fed animal fats
- Palm oils
- Vegetable oils removed from original source

When it comes to fat, the key is *caution*. Too much of even *good* fat will make your body fat. Of all the food categories, fats have more calories per unit. Need I say more?

Combining Fats with Carbohydrates and Proteins

▶ Body by God Owner's Tip: Get Skinny on Fat

The concept of eating fat-free is not only unhealthy, but it may also cause you to get fat. Good fats such as those found in flaxseed, olives, and fish help the body mobilize stored fats. Additionally, the body must take in fat to stay adept at absorbing and utilizing it. Adding small to moderate amounts of good fats to healthy, low-fat Food by God will help the Body by God to function better and actually make it leaner.

The Body by God needs some fat in its diet. When combining fats with carbohydrates and/or proteins, you should be extra careful. Eating carbohydrates all by themselves causes huge amounts of sugar to be dumped into your body's system, making the pancreas put out large amounts of insulin to control the rising blood sugar levels. Ironically, your body will want even more carbohydrates and sugar in response to the lowering blood sugar levels created by the insulin's rush to the rescue. It's true: eating carbohydrates creates a hunger for more carbohydrates! The trick is to add small amounts of fats or small amounts of proteins to carbohydrate-heavy meals, creating a more gradual carbohydrate-digestion speed.

To slow the rise in blood sugar (and consequently, the excessive production of insulin by the pancreas), add a small amount of a healthy fat, or a small serving of protein, or a very small serving of both when eating a carbohydrate. For example: one egg (protein) with oatmeal (carbohydrate) sweetened with a teaspoon of almond butter (good fat), toast with extra-virgin olive oil drizzled on it, and ground flaxseed sprinkled on a sweet potato. (If this sounds like a weird combination to you, don't knock it until you've tried it!)

You could also try adding a moderate amount of fats to a larger serving of proteins, such as: salmon (protein/good fat) Caesar salad with avocados (good fat) and olives (good fat), or chicken, cashews, and broccoli stir-fried in extra-virgin olive oil, and a one-egg-yolk/four-egg-white omelet cooked in a skillet greased with coconut oil.

On the *Don't Do This!* side of the menu are pizza, linguini Alfredo, donuts, pancakes, hash browns, cookies, bread and butter, and a loaded potato. This type of meal with large amounts of fat and larger servings of carbohydrates will make you fat. Period.

And then there's the *heart-explosion meal*. It's too many fats, carbohydrates, and proteins together, causing a great increase in pulse rate, blood pressure, and cholesterol. An example would be a steak-and-cheese sub, eggs and pancakes with butter and syrup, or a cheeseburger and French fries. How unbalanced can a meal get?

Back to Basics

The way the majority of people eat today is dangerous to the Body by God because it produces high levels of acid, altering the basic pH environment necessary for the tissues and organs to survive and thrive. A highly acidic environment in the body literally burns the cells themselves. This acidic environment is also directly related to issues such as bone loss, fibromyalgia, muscle problems, and degeneration from arthritis. When we overconsume foods that produce acid on a regular basis, we literally deluge our kidneys with an excessive acid level that is more than they can handle well. This situation causes the body to neutralize the acid by pulling calcium phosphate and calcium carbonate from the bones. Obviously this is not good for the bones.

The leading food categories that produce acid can be found on the Food by Man list and include commercial dairy products, flour, sugar, caffeine, and all animal products. Whole grains and fruits are slightly acid-producing as well, even though they are Food by God, so follow the Body by God Un-Diet guidelines to be sure you eat them at the proper time and with the right complementary foods.

Vegetables do exceptionally well at producing more of the basic environment necessary for optimum health in the Body by God. You can help stabilize the acids in your system and promote healing in your joints and other organs by eating all the vegetables you can. Other foods that help correct acid imbalance are almonds, avocados, and flaxseed. Drinking a great deal of clean water is also extremely important for a healthy environment. Speaking of water . . .

Water

The Body by God can survive for weeks without food, but after a few days of water deprivation, all of the body's systems begin to malfunction. The Body by God is mostly water, and the health of each of your body's cells depends upon the quality of the fluids in your diet. It stands to reason that if you drink poor-quality water, or coffee, or soda that the water in your body will be contaminated with chemicals, additives, and other pollutants not intended for human consumption. Your body needs pure, clean water to continuously flush out the poisons and acids you are consuming and producing each day.

You'd really have to work at it to consume too much water, but simply ignoring your body's need for water and plenty of it works against your health and makes it harder for your body to operate at peak efficiency.

▶ Tip: Drinking Water Promotes Good Health

The combination of drinking plenty of water and focusing on a more basic diet will help in recovering or sparing the bones and joints of your Body by God. Always remember: a dry joint is an unhappy joint.

A word about pH: pH is a measure of acidity and alkalinity in the body. A healthy balance at the middle of the pH scale would be a reading of 7.0. Anything higher than that means your body is too alkaline; anything less than that means your body is too acidic. Any imbalance in your pH makes your body try to correct the situation. You can improve your body's chance to achieve a balance of pH 7 by drinking more water, which will also rehydrate your body, keeping it healthy for both you and your baby.

Nutrients by God

Vitamins, minerals, amino acids, antioxidants, and all nutrients known to man (and also those only God knows about) are the basic foundation of the Body by God. All of these nutrients are necessary for a healthy body and a happy life and can be found in Food by God. I cannot stress enough the need to obtain these nutrients from foods that are as close as possible to their natural state—untampered with by man. When fruits and vegetables are processed by cooking, pasteurization, or other refining processes, they mutate into a different product that hinders the body in absorbing the nutrients.

The synergy of the essential elements of a Food by God (or *nutrient communion*, as it is called), means that you need to eat whole foods that provide not only the nutrient you want (vitamin A, for example), but also the other elements *within* that food that *balance* the makeup of that food so your Body by God can do a complete job of processing the nutrient (beta-carotene in a carrot, for example). Simply put, the best way to provide vitamin A for your body is by eating a carrot, not by taking a synthetic vitamin pill. Without nutrient communion, or the synergy found in whole foods, vitamins isolated in supplements can even do great harm.

▶ Nutrient Tip: A Little Extra Help

Nutrient supplements are critical due to the significant unlikelihood that anyone will eat enough of the right foods on a regular basis to obtain all the nutrients necessary for good health. But supplements are just that: they are *supplemental* or *in addition to* taking in the right nutrients in the form of food. Supplements cannot replace the real nutrients found only in God-made food.

I believe it is necessary to take high-quality vitamin, mineral, and omega-3 oil supplements on a daily basis. You should purchase these from a natural health-care provider or a health food store. A lifetime of improper eating habits cannot be undone in a couple of days. You will need to make a commitment to yourself, your baby, and to God if you intend to live to the fullest the life He has given you.

11 | The Un-Diet Food Guide

The truth is out: diets do not work! In fact, they cause suffering, can even be dangerous to your health, and almost always leave you right where you started—or worse. Diets are not normal (and certainly not preferred) ways of eating. They usually restrict one type of food or another, when it's really the *balance* of nutrients that the body craves.

On some diets, *some* people can lose weight. But what have you really accomplished if you lose ten pounds in forty-eight hours by drinking somebody's idea of a juice cocktail? You may weigh less, but you are not healthier. Yes, I lost weight when I was on my *diet*. But my diet was not eating at *all* and was very, very unhealthy.

On the Un-Diet, there is no calorie counting, no beginning, and no end. You just learn to eat better and keep getting better at it. It's eating the way God intended you to eat, so He'll help you do it. Unlike other diets, the Un-Diet works for everyone. The Un-Diet brings your highs and lows into balance, making a difference in how you feel and in your energy level.

Don't be fooled: no diet can heal your body. But given the right tools, the Body by God can heal itself. To heal my body from my years of unhealthy eating, I needed the Un-Diet—a way of eating in order to give my Body by God optimum health from the Food by God I consume. Basically, it's eating the right foods at the right times and in the right combinations.

As I stated before, this doesn't happen overnight, because you have to create new habits. But the sooner you move toward eating the way God intended, the sooner you move toward a healthier body that can bounce back more quickly.

The Un-Diet can remove the obstacles that keep your body from being able to heal itself. It only makes sense: stop putting toxins into the body, and it will be able to concentrate on giving you the power you need to fulfill your God-inspired destiny. The U.S. Army has a slogan: Be All You Can Be. That's *apropos* for the Un-Diet too. It allows your body to be all it can be physically, and that spills over into the emotional and spiritual arenas as well.

The Three Simple Steps to Un-Dieting
1. Begin adding Food by God.
2. Begin reducing Food by Man.
3. Follow the Food Guide.

In my practice I have seen excellent results in people who have eaten very few (or even none) of the Food by God choices but have followed the Food Guide's recommendations regarding *when* to eat the different categories of foods.

▶ Un-Diet Tip: Subtraction by Addition
The perfect Un-Diet is 80 to 90 percent Food by God (so only 10 to 20 percent Food by Man), and eating the right foods at the right time of day according to the Food Guide.

The great news is that if you apply any of the three steps to Un-Dieting, you will see marked improvement. The key to the Un-Diet is to focus on adding good foods, not taking food away.

12 | The Body by God Un-Diet

Now the question is, what to eat and when? Mornings are when you need the most energy, so carbohydrates should be on the menu. That's also the time of day when your system should have used up whatever you ate at the evening meal or later, so your Body by God will need fuel when you get up. Eating carbohydrates in the morning gives you all day to burn them off. They will also provide high-quality fiber that your body easily utilizes and is full of vitamins and minerals. *One word of caution:* don't eat too many carbohydrates because it could work against you. Keep bread, sugars, and cereals to a single serving.

> *Tell them, "In the evening you will have meat and in the morning you will be stuffed with bread, and you shall know that I am Jehovah your God."*
> —Exodus 16:12 TLB

When I was first learning how to eat healthy using the Un-Diet, I began to feel much better. As a result, I exercised more and decided I would try to run a marathon (twenty-six miles). The most I had ever run before was five or six miles. My eating habits were still not perfect, and I tried to run without eating breakfast or on just a cup of coffee. I just couldn't do it. Needless to say, I hadn't transformed my life or my eating habits enough to run that marathon, but it didn't stop me from forging ahead. Instead it gave me more motivation to continue my quest for health. Eventually I learned that I needed to fuel my body in the morning so that I could run more than forty-five minutes at a time.

▶ **Tip: Like Carbs? Eat Them in the A.M.**

If you do nothing else but follow the Food Guide, the morning is the best time for bread, pastries, and pizza. All have an overwhelming amount of carbohydrates that require as much of the day as possible to burn.

Preferred Morning Foods

Fruit

Your best source of fiber, vitamins, and minerals in the morning is fruit. Fruit is one of God's perfect foods. It is best to consume fruit only in the morning, and it is best to eat fruit first. If a lot of other foods are already in the food processing system, the fruit will not pass through the digestive process effectively. Fruit sugars caught in the system have the potential to produce a harmful, yeast-producing effect on body chemistry.

The best fruits include grapefruit, figs, tomatoes, avocados, plums, nectarines, apples, pears, pineapple, currants, oranges, tangerines, berries, and melons eaten by themselves without other fruits or foods.

▶ **Un-Diet Tip:**

Eat fruit only in the morning, and only one or two pieces.

Unprocessed Whole Grains and Sweeteners

Oats, grits, cream of whole wheat, puffed brown rice, quinoa, cream of brown rice, and jasmine or basmati rice are all good examples of whole grain breakfast foods. The less refined and chemically treated, the better. Oats are typically the easiest to obtain in their most unrefined form.

To sweeten and flavor these foods, don't use cow's milk, sugar, or butter. Use instead almond butter (tastes just as good or better than peanut butter, and it is healthier), almond or rice milk, fruit, unrefined honey, or maple syrup. This allows this carbohydrate breakfast to be very user-friendly and relatively Food by Man–free.

Less-Preferred Morning Foods

Chemical-Free Refined Foods and Sweeteners

Breads and cereals are popular, easy morning foods. The problem with these products is that they are refined, man-made, and very concentrated carbohydrates. Typical refined products contain dangerous additives, preservatives, sugars, and hydrogenated oils and are not made from whole grains.

If you are going to eat refined foods, such as breads and cereals, for breakfast, it is important that they not contain chemicals and preservatives and that they be made up of whole grains still containing some fiber and nutrients. Sweeten or flavor with almond butter, fresh fruit juice, maple syrup, unrefined honey, or raw organic butter.

▶ Tip: Best Breakfast Choices

Foods made with oat, brown rice, buckwheat, spelt, or millet flour, live sprouted grains, and quinoa. Although these may sound foreign to you, you can find them all at local health food stores and bakeries, and they taste great.

Use Non-Cow Milk

Use almond or rice milk instead of cow's milk.

Reduced-Carbohydrate / High-Protein Breakfast

This is also a good plan for someone who has trouble digesting fruits and grains, is significantly overweight, has other digestive troubles, or has blood-sugar difficulties. Cutting back the portion of carbohydrates and adding more quality protein and good fat will help to control blood-sugar fluctuation. Reducing carbohydrates in the morning is also a good idea if you took in too many carbohydrates the day or evening before.

It is important to consume the highest-quality protein source available in the morning. Since proteins and carbohydrates do not digest well together, you should eat proteins with only a small amount of carbohydrates. The morning is not a good time to start a food war in the body.

An egg is unrefined and the highest-level protein source available. Pork and pork products that Americans typically consume during breakfast are heavily refined, toxic, and classic Food by Man. I do not recommend them as the protein of choice.

Acid-reducing vegetables are good to eat with animal proteins. Therefore, an ideal protein breakfast would be a vegetable omelet using three to four egg whites and one egg yolk, without any or just a small amount of other food from the carbohydrate category. Cook the eggs using olive or coconut oil.

When you add a carbohydrate to a protein breakfast, make sure to use *only* one serving of the most complete grain possible; for example, one serving of oatmeal or one slice of whole grain bread.

Morning Beverages

Water, Fresh-Squeezed Juices, Herb Tea, Almond Milk

The morning is an important time for high-quality liquids. Since you have not had anything to drink for several hours, the body is dehydrated. When dehydrated, the body needs liquids, and it will quickly absorb whatever you drink into the tissues.

You do not want to bathe your organ cells in coffee, tea, and soda, but in great fluids such as water or fresh, unrefined, nonpasteurized fruit or vegetable juice. You should consume fruit juice, like all fruits, on as empty a stomach as possible.

It is important to drink two to four glasses of pure water throughout the morning. Since the body is depleted of nutrients at this time and thus geared up for heavy absorption, the morning is also a good time for high-quality vitamin and mineral supplements.

Hot herbal tea or hot rice or almond milk is a good alternative to coffee or regular tea in the mornings.

Late-Morning Snacks

In the late morning, it is important to not add too many more carbohydrates. Try adding one piece of fruit, one more serving of whole grains, or changing away from carbohydrates to vegetables, or eggs and vegetables.

Condiments

Fats

Ground flaxseed, olive oil, coconut oil, walnuts, almonds, and almond butter.

Seasonings

Butter Buds (replacement food for butter), cinnamon, maple syrup, molasses, and honey.

Preferred Morning Carbohydrates Options

Option #1

One piece or serving of fruit or glass of freshly squeezed fruit juice. (Drink fresh juice only. Pasteurized juice has too much sugar, and its nutrients are damaged or destroyed during processing. If fresh fruit juice is not possible, cut pasteurized juice in half with water, or cut it out all together.)

Later or Option #2

Hot whole grain cereal (oats, grits, cream of wheat, cream of rice, quinoa) or brown, basmati, or jasmine rice or rice cake. (You can mix these different grains together to create variety in your hot cereal or to find a way you like to eat it.)

Add: ground flaxseed for good fat, almond butter, or sliced almonds.

Sweeten with: rice or almond milk, honey, and/or fruit if you did not eat fruit earlier in the morning.

Condiments: Butter Buds, cinnamon.

Less-Preferred Options

Option #3

All natural, no-chemical, whole grain cereal that is sweetened with fruit, honey, or unsweetened with almond or rice milk.

Add: ground flaxseed and/or sliced almonds.

Option #4

All-natural, whole grain, chemical-free bread with almond butter or small amount of extra-virgin olive oil and one whole egg.

High Proteins/Low Carbohydrates Options

Option #5

Three- to four-egg-white and one-egg-yolk vegetable omelet; no additional carbohydrates.

Option #6

Three to four egg whites and one egg yolk with one piece of whole grain bread, or one serving of Option #2 or #3.

Late-Morning snack

One piece of fruit, one serving of oats, vegetables, or vegetable omelet.

 A Perfect Way to Combine Your Morning Options

- Eat fruit or drink fresh fruit juice first and then, later in the morning, choose from Options #1–4.

- Follow good food-combining rules by eating a carbohydrate and good fat only at breakfast (e.g., oatmeal, banana, ground flaxseed, and almond butter); then, two to four hours later, eat a protein (two- to four-egg-white omelets).

- If time or convenience is an issue, choose #2, #3, or #4 and keep a piece of fruit with you for a snack later. You can save oatmeal and rice and bring them with you in airtight containers.

▲ ▲ ▲

Midday

Moderate to Low Carbohydrates / Moderate Proteins / Low to Moderate Fats

The key to a balanced diet is recognizing the fact that not all meals are created equally. For instance, in the morning, carbohydrates were important to replenish your power stores to face the long day ahead. Now, as the afternoon approaches, lunch is a different matter. You don't need as many carbohydrates in the afternoon and most likely have sugar in your blood left over from your morning meal. There is now less day left, and so, therefore, less sugar you need to burn.

Additionally, you have now used your body to some degree. Therefore, you do not just need power foods; you need some food for healing and repair. You now need some protein.

If you have a physically demanding job or exercise later in the day, you will need to eat some extra carbohydrates at midday or in the early evening to provide yourself with the extra power boost. If you have an increased need to lose weight, decrease blood pressure or cholesterol points, reduce carbohydrates at midday as you do in the evening.

Where breakfast was a carbohydrate-focused meal with little or no protein, lunch is going to contain moderate to low amounts of carbohydrates and moderate to high amounts of protein. Morning was time for fruit, one of God's perfect foods. Afternoon and evening are times for God's other perfect food, vegetables. Lots of them.

If Following the Un-Diet Food Guide Rules Only

Because of their high carbohydrate content, try to get breads and pastas out of the way at lunch. As in the morning, continue to avoid heavy doses of protein such as red meat or large servings of chicken or fish.

Preferred Midday Carbohydrates

The best midday carbohydrates are medium- to small-sized portions of those foods that look the way they did when they were still in the ground. The best lunchtime carbohydrate foods are starchy carbohydrates (sweet potatoes, potatoes, corn, peas, squash) and beans. Next on the list is brown, basmati, or jasmine rice, or other whole grains.

Less-Preferred Midday Carbohydrates

The next-best choices for carbohydrates at midday are chemical-free, whole grain breads and pastas. While still somewhat refined and high in carbohydrates, they have nutritional value and are not as refined as white bread, white pasta, and wheat bread that contain additives.

Totally refined carbohydrate foods such as pasta, bread, and white rice cannot be properly digested and have a lot of carbohydrates per serving. These will be more likely to sit in your intestine, cause a spike and dip in your blood sugar, and make you tired in the afternoon.

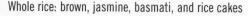

List of Best Grains*

Whole rice: brown, jasmine, basmati, and rice cakes
- Whole grain breads: live-sprouted grains such as millet, spelt, rye, brown rice, buckwheat, soy, and gluten-free
- Whole grain pasta: rice, corn, spelt, and wheat

*See Whole Grain Rule (page 94)

▲ ▲ ▲

Preferred Midday Fats

Use olive oil, ground flaxseed, flaxseed oil, and avocado with your midday carbohydrates as your source of healthy fats and to control blood sugar changes.

Preferred Midday Proteins

Light Proteins

Because proteins do not combine well with carbohydrates and are difficult to break down and eliminate, midday proteins should be light, lean, and in medium portions. Good examples are four egg whites with one egg yolk, four ounces of tuna, fish, chicken breast, or turkey breast.

Nonanimal Proteins

Beans contain carbohydrates and proteins and combine well with whole grains as an extremely healthy, nonanimal protein lunch with only slightly more than moderate levels of carbohydrates. Good nonanimal protein sources include lentils, lima beans, and unprocessed soybeans.

Heavier Protein, Low Carbohydrates

If you eat a larger portion (six to ten ounces or more) of an animal product or a heavier protein, eat it with a salad and vegetables and very little or no dense carbohydrates such as breads, pasta, rice, or starchy vegetables.

Meal-Splitting

A great idea for getting the carbohydrates and protein you need during the midday, without causing problems by combining too much of the two together, is to split up these afternoon meals.

Eat a heavier carbohydrate meal first. Then, two to three hours later, eat a protein meal or protein, then carbohydrates. This is known as *meal-splitting*.

Meal-splitting works particularly well if you have a physically demanding job or compete in athletics later in the day. You can have a typical medium-protein, medium-carbohydrate lunch so as not to combine too much of the two and then, two to three hours later, add some more good carbohydrates to give you a power boost when you need it later in the day.

Condiments

Condiments and spices are good for flavoring natural foods. Limit fat use when consuming large to moderate amounts of carbohydrates. It is important at midday meals to use only moderate amounts of healthy fats and to limit or eliminate altogether animal fats found in dairy products and high-fat meats such as red meat, dark-meat chicken, dark-meat turkey, and pork.

Use olive oil for cooking and olive oil and lemon for dressings. Flavor using hot sauces, tamari, mustards, and other condiments that contain no chemicals, bad fats, or sugars.

Good seasonings include basil, curry, dill, garlic, ginger, horse-radish, mint, miso, mustard, paprika, parsley, rosemary, soy, tamari, tarragon, and thyme.

Late-Afternoon/Early-Evening Snacks

In the late afternoon, your snacks should consist of medium carbo-hydrates, or vegetables with protein.

Raw and roasted nuts and seeds are a great afternoon or early evening snack. Walnuts contain omega-3 fats, and almonds are in the acid-reducing food category, so they are the most recommended along with raw pumpkin and sunflower seeds. Soaking raw nuts and seeds for several hours makes them more palatable and easier to digest. Another good snack at this time is vegetables with only a light protein.

You should limit intake of nuts and seeds unless you are follow-ing the Un-Diet rule of only vegetables and proteins for dinner. Nuts and seeds are high in fat and so should not be combined with carbo-hydrates or proteins. (See Combining Fats with Carbohydrates and Proteins on page 99.)

Midday Beverages

Beverages consumed toward the middle of your day should consist of only pure water, fresh vegetable juices, or herbal teas that are unsweet-ened or lightly sweetened with rice milk, almond milk, or honey.

Preferred Midday Options

Option #1
Medium to small amount of starchy carbohydrates such as

sweet potatoes, peas, squash, or potatoes with vegetables, salads, and light protein: eggs, tuna, or small portion of fish, turkey, or chicken breast.

Option #2

Brown, basmati, or jasmine rice.

Less-Preferred Midday Options

Option #3

Whole-grain pasta or additive-free, whole grain bread with light protein.

Option #4

Vegetarian: Brown, basmati, or jasmine rice or whole grain pasta or additive-free whole grain bread with beans.

Option #5

Low Carbohydrate: Vegetables, salad, and larger amount of good protein (eggs, chicken, turkey, or fish).

▶ Tip: Stretch Out Your Meals

Remember that you can always split protein and carbohydrates into two meals. For example: vegetable, salad, and tuna at noon, and then a sweet potato at 2:00 PM, or the other way around.

Evening Foods

Low Carbohydrates / High Proteins / Moderate to High Fats

When you go to sleep at night, your body begins its natural repair process. It uses protein for building and repair. So the best time for eating concentrated animal protein is at night.

In the evening, you must be careful to avoid concentrated

carbohydrates, either altogether or as much as possible. Not long after dinner you are typically going to go to bed. Therefore, you don't want to eat a lot of carbohydrates and go right to bed because you will not have used all that sugar power. *Try to stick to protein and vegetables only.*

The other reason to just say no to concentrated carbohydrates at night is that this is a heavy protein meal. A lot of protein and carbohydrates mixed together will wreak havoc on your fuel processing system all night long, making it hard to sleep and even harder to get up.

If Following the Un-Diet Food Guide Rules Only

Red meat, pork, and cheese eaters would do best to eat these foods only at night and without any carbohydrates other than vegetables and salads. Avoid bread, pasta, potatoes, and rice with these foods as there is not much use for carbohydrates at night, and high-protein, high-fat items such as these do not combine well with carbohydrates.

Preferred Evening Foods

Just Animal Protein and Vegetables

High-quality, lean animal proteins including fish, chicken breast, and turkey breast are your best choices. All animal products come with problems inherent with their use. As a result, protein choices should be extremely varied throughout the week.

Again, due to their ability to help balance out the acidic effect of animal proteins, their high vitamin and mineral content, and the fact that they do not contain many carbohydrates, vegetables should be eaten with the evening meal.

Less-Preferred Evening Foods

If you eat carbohydrates other than vegetables in the evening, avoid the overly dense, refined varieties such as breads and pastas, and stick to the more moderate, natural ones such as peas, corn, sweet potatoes, potatoes, and whole grain rice.

 ## Good Evening Proteins

Examples include chicken breast, turkey breast, tuna, grouper, mahimahi, sardines, mackerel, halibut, cod, rainbow trout, swordfish, sturgeon, whitefish, and lean beef.

Vary all animal intake due to toxicity. Free-range, organic, grass- and/or vegetable-fed beef, chicken, and eggs are less toxic and have good fats, so I recommend them if you can afford, find, or raise them on your own.

Evening Snacks

Snacks during the late evening should consist of low- to zero-carbohydrate foods such as raw nuts and seeds, vegetables, and animal proteins.

Evening Beverages

Beverages consumed toward the end of your day should consist of only pure water and fresh vegetable juices.

Condiments

Use extra-virgin olive oil for cooking and olive oil and lemon for dressings. Flavor using hot sauces, tamari, mustards, and other condiments that contain no chemicals, bad fats, or sugars. Good seasonings include basil, curry, dill, garlic, ginger, horseradish, mint, miso, mustard, paprika, parsley, rosemary, soy, tamari, tarragon, and thyme.

Preferred Evening Options

Option #1

Full serving of fish, turkey, chicken, or lean beef with *large servings* of vegetables and salad.

Less-Preferred Evening Options

Option #2

Fish, turkey, or chicken with vegetables and small serving of starchy carbohydrate or brown, basmati, or jasmine rice.

Option #3

Vegetarian: Small serving of brown, basmati, or jasmine rice with beans and vegetables.

Evening Snacks

Vegetables and/or more protein (low carbohydrates).

Special Considerations

Some people need more power during the day; for example, people who have physically demanding jobs and athletes. These groups of people should eat more Food by God from the carbohydrate category. Meal-splitting is the best way to space out the power foods; the body can absorb only so much at one time. An extra carbohydrate meal in late morning and late afternoon is a good idea.

If you are trying to build more muscle or strength, adding more protein and carbohydrates might help. Protein *builds* muscle; carbohydrates *spare* muscle. Again, meal-splitting is great for adding more protein, particularly at these times: late morning (protein), late afternoon (protein/carbohydrates), and after dinner (protein).

Athletes and people who burn up a lot of carbohydrates, in particular, should eat more carbohydrates right after their sessions. The rest of us can gain more power not by eating more food, but by eating more correctly.

Children and the Un-Diet

You hold your children's futures in your hands as you feed them. Their physical well-being is paramount in your mind, of course, and if you have read this far, you are serious about giving them the proper nutritional start in life. While you are nursing your newborn, your own nutrition is vital to that of your baby. What you have eaten, he or she also eats through your breast milk. Choose your Food by God well!

Children are prime candidates for a Food by God lifestyle because their bodies are just beginning to be formed. It is never too early to introduce good nutrition to them. Junk food and fast food are filled with chemicals and toxins and have no place in the diet of a child—of *any* age.

We've all seen toddlers and young children who have one bout of sickness or infection right after another. You can avoid much, if not all, of that by following the Body by God principles as you introduce solid foods and then mealtimes into your child's diet.

13 | Weight Loss for Bouncing Back

After you give birth to your child, the first thing you want to do is get your figure back to where it was before you became pregnant—or better. During pregnancy you eat for at least two people, not just to nourish your own body, so the weight begins to add up. Then the baby is born and suddenly you have lost about ten to fifteen pounds. What about the rest of it? How can you get rid of it, preferably by Saturday night when your husband has invited you out on your first postpartum date and you want to wear that hot little black dress you haven't been able to get into for nine months?

You've probably already figured out that Food by Man is *not* the answer! But Food by God is your first line of defense. I don't use the word *defense* lightly. Your body is used to eating, and eating pretty much *when* and *what* you craved during your pregnancy. It's been said that it takes three months to establish a habit that will last a lifetime. You've just been through *nine* months of less-than-great eating habits. It's a temptation to just throw up your hands and give in. You're hungry all the time, you're tired all the time, and you just don't have the energy to fight it. But yes, you *do*.

You get the energy to fight the weight off from the same source your energy to birth a healthy baby came from: God. He's the one who gave you the strength to care for yourself and your baby while you were waiting to deliver. He's the one who wants to help you care for your baby's growing body (and weight gain) at the same time you care for your shrinking body (and weight loss). After all, He created both of you, He loves both of you, and He knows what both of you need. He's also ready and more than willing to work right through every challenge with each of you.

So there's no need for you to go it alone when it comes to getting your figure back after delivery. Be honest: you need all the help you can get! It's going to take commitment, determination, sweat, and tears, but you can do it—with God's help. All you have to do is ask Him, and He'll be there through every deep knee-bend, every ab crunch, and every defeated temptation to eat half a dozen chocolate donuts. Together, you can get that prepregnancy body back—maybe even better than it was.

Food by God is clean and efficient fuel for your Body by God. Unlike Food by Man, it doesn't pollute your body and leave unused deposits of fat on your hips and other unmentionable places. Actually it helps eliminate some of what Food by Man leaves in your body.

The Un-Diet is what God intended us to eat. If you follow the Un-Diet Food Guide and choose foods from the Food by God lists, your body will begin to move toward its ideal weight for your frame. But there *are* some things you can do to help move things along.

The following choices will create the fastest changes:

- Do away with heavy carbohydrates such as bread, pasta, and other flour products.
- Do not eat any carbohydrate-rich foods after your midday meal. Eat only green vegetables as carbohydrates in the late afternoon and evening (as seen in the Un-Diet Food Guide).
- Drink more water and vegetable juices and less of any other beverages, and cut out any stimulant drinks such as coffee, soda, or tea.
- Massively limit—or abolish—Food by Man.

Weight-Loss Warning and Recommendation

To avoid the failures that typically accompany restricting foods, just follow the Body by God Un-Diet closely and add more movement (follow the Exercise by God program on pages 144–147). More movement allows you to burn extra fat and calories so that you may lose weight.

▲ ▲ ▲

Start the Un-Diet plan, be patient, and move your Body by God more often. This will not only speed up the weight-loss process, but it's also just plain good for you.

A Word About Metabolism

Metabolism refers to how many calories your body burns whether you are resting or working. Hormone levels play a part in determining your metabolism rate and the intensity of the level your cells are working at; using up your power (burning calories) figures into it as well.

I'm sure you've heard people who are overweight say their condition is due to a glandular problem called PGS (Poor Genetic Syndrome). The truth is that some people may have a genetic or inherited tendency to store fat and burn fewer calories, but most of us increase or decrease our metabolism rates by the choices we make. It stands to reason that if you eat more calories than you use, you gain weight. If you burn more calories than you eat, you lose weight. Following the Un-Diet guidelines and moving more will do more to get your prepregnancy body back than all the genetics in your family tree.

If you feel stuck with the body you have, you *can* get unstuck. It takes a daily commitment. (Sometimes it takes a minute-by-minute commitment!) It takes knowledge (which you're gaining right now), work, and prayer. But you *can* do it! I believe in you, and God does too.

The Truth Behind Metabolism

The speed and efficiency at which your body burns fat and calories are determined more by the way you live your life and less by your genetics. Movement, multiple fuelings, and eating foods at the right time of day that God designed for the human digestive system all speed up or normalize the metabolism and cause the Body by God to find or maintain its ideal ratio of loosely packed muscle to tightly packed muscle.

▲ ▲ ▲

14 | Rules for Better Fueling

If the Body by God principles and the Un-Diet guidelines are new to you, then you're probably thinking you'll never be able to make the shift to this new and healthier lifestyle. Please believe me when I say I'm not advocating that you take your existing diet and deposit it at the town dump. I know from my own experience that changing your eating lifestyle can be very hard.

Rules for better fueling will help you make the transition and change your eating lifestyle gradually. Thousands of people have followed these rules and are enjoying good health and thinner bodies. You can do it too.

The Addition Rule:
Instead of Eliminating the Bad, Add the Good

To make a lasting change in your eating lifestyle, make it slowly. Most people eat, but what they eat does not provide the proper nourishment for their bodies, leaving them overfed but undernourished. Much of what they consume is high-calorie food with no nutritive value.

If lunch for you means a soda and a candy bar, try adding an apple. Psychologically, if you are told to eliminate something from your diet, you immediately want it even more. You *love* that candy bar, right? You feel deprived if you try denying yourself the pleasure of its company. So don't. Instead *add* Food by God a little at a time, and someday soon you'll surprise yourself by choosing the apple instead of the candy bar, and a glass of rice milk instead of the soda. Your cravings will change for the better.

The Replacement Rule:
Substitute Something from a Health Food Store That Is Similar to the Form and Taste of a Nutrition-Devoid Food by Man You Crave

You can get addicted to foods such as pizza, ice cream, sugared cereal, and fast foods. Addictions get in the way of making healthy food choices. Caving in to cravings is a normal human condition. The Replacement Rule helps you feel increasingly satisfied with healthier choices until the cravings are conquered.

Replacement Foods

Craving/Addiction	Replacement Food
Pizza: store-bought	Whole grain pizza with all-natural or homemade sauce and low-fat, un-refined cheese
Ice cream	Nondairy, low-fat alternative (e.g., Rice Dream)
Sugary, refined cereal	One of the many health-food, whole grain cereals with rice or almond milk
Sugar	Honey, fresh fruit juice, unrefined maple syrup, molasses, brown rice syrup
Salt, MSG	Healthy spices and condiments
Rich desserts	Whole grain, nondairy, chemical-free, low-fat or honey- or fruit-sweetened treats

| Fast-food burger | Lean, homemade all-beef burger, lean turkey burger, or veggie burger |
| Cheese | Low-fat, unrefined cheese and nondairy cheese, such as rice cheese |

The Ten-Point Reduction Rule:
If You Can Reduce a Food Craving, You'll
Have More Power Over Your Eating Decisions

Bo Derek is a "ten." On a scale of one to ten, your cravings are a ten, but they won't leave you with a gorgeous body like Bo Derek's! If you could get your cravings down from a ten to a seven or eight, they would be somewhat controlled. If you could get them down even lower, perhaps to a three or four, you could eventually eliminate them.

Reducing the intensity of the craving (whether it's that first cup of coffee in the morning or an ice-cream cone every summer evening) allows you to eventually say no to it. While you're getting to that point, when the craving hits with a passion, reach for a piece of fruit or something fat-free or naturally sweetened.

The Vacation Food Rule:
You Don't Cave If You Crave

You didn't get where you are in your eating habits overnight. It took years of constant struggle to achieve the dubious proficiency of choosing the wrong foods that you now consume. The good news is that it probably will not take years to undo the poor choices and establish a healthier eating lifestyle. Given half a chance, the Body by God will naturally gravitate toward more healthy decisions. But it doesn't have that chance when you constantly stuff it with poor ones.

While on your way to that healthier lifestyle, it's perfectly permissible to give yourself a break. No one (not even my husband and I) can be 100 percent disciplined 100 percent of the time. The

Vacation Food Rule is all about giving yourself a break as you work toward your goal. Giving in to a craving or eating poor choices from the Food by Man list of foods is an integral part of the Un-Diet plan. Planning a vacation is half the fun of taking one.

If you're addicted to pizza, for example, this rule allows you to choose to eat pizza once a week, for example, Saturday night. All week long you can look forward to pizza night. The anticipation gets you through the week, helping you make better choices from the Food by God list for the six days leading up to Saturday.

Some cravings are harder to beat than others. With this Vacation Food Rule, however, you can lower the craving's intensity and eventually eliminate it. I personally love sweets, and if I eat them I try to do the Vacation Food Rule and get back on track the next day; once I start eating sweets, it's hard to stop. One trick I've learned is that if I crave sweets, I will buy only *one* serving and finish it. When it's done, it's gone, and it can't continue to tempt me. I find that if there is some left the next day, it's hard not to eat it.

One of my favorite places back home was a bakery. I grew up on its cake and icing. When I went home to visit, my family ordered me cake as a treat. Unfortunately, I ate it for breakfast, lunch, and dinner every day until it was gone. Now I tell my family not to order me a cake, but instead buy me one piece of it. If you just have enough for a vacation *day* instead of a vacation *week*, it really helps.

The Food Dress-Up Rule:
Add Taste and Eye Appeal
with Healthy Add-Ins

Americans have desensitized their taste buds. The fact is that the additives, sugars, salts, and fats that are omnipresent in Foods by Man have dulled our God-given sense of taste. Food by God (natural foods) has incredible taste on its own; we just aren't able to perceive it anymore.

Oatmeal, for example, is one of the best things on the Food by God list; however, it has a bland taste all by itself. Try adding fruits, nuts, granola, or even small amounts of other healthy cereals for a different taste that will make your mouth sit up and pay attention.

The Stay Full Rule: Don't Get Too Hungry

Hunger triggers one response in all humans: *I've got to get something to eat!* Because we're busy, we grab the first available thing to put into our mouths to stop the hunger pangs. Usually (especially if we are not at home where we keep healthy foods) that's a Food by Man because it's handy at every corner convenience store and fast-food place. If you have a job that keeps you on the road, it's hard when hunger hits. It takes *planning* to eat healthy snacks and meals, and that takes time. Most of us don't have (or take) the time to plan ahead, so we end up choosing Food by Man on the run. This is not good.

Eating regular meals from Food by God at the proper times of the day for those food categories maintains a healthy balance of nourishment and satisfaction. Skipping meals creates an emergency situation where we eat anything within reach. Don't let yourself get too hungry. Plan for hunger attacks and prepare for them with Food by God choices.

The Multiple Feedings Rule: Eat Several Smaller, Lighter, Healthier Meals Throughout the Day

Weight loss produces hunger while your body is adjusting to your new way of eating. It's inevitable. We've all been taught to eat three square meals a day. It's healthier to eat six smaller, well-chosen meals a day. Smaller meals digest more easily, provide a sustained level of energy, and increase the metabolic rate of the Body by God.

I have a friend who fuels her body about every three hours. She rises early (5 or 6 AM), has her breakfast, and works in her home office until around 9 AM, when she notices her stomach feels empty and her energy is beginning to lag. She has a healthy snack and then works until noon when she has lunch. By three she's ready for another snack. She has dinner at 6 PM, and then a healthy snack just before bedtime around 9 PM. This works well for her and is a very healthy lifestyle.

When she has to travel for her work, she prepares plenty of Food by God snacks to take in the car. She has gradually weaned herself off Food by Man over the past six months and has lost thirty pounds. Her blood pressure has gone down enough that her doctor has decreased the medication dosage originally prescribed. Her cholesterol level was 276 when she began making changes in her diet and exercise—or rather, the lack of it! After three months she decreased the total cholesterol level to 204. She has walked two miles, three times a week during this six-month period as well. She has dropped two dress sizes. What does she say about this lifestyle change for the better? "I'll never go back to what or when I was eating before! I feel too good without it!"

You don't have to start applying these rules all at once. Try one a week and see what a difference it makes in how you feel. If one of them just doesn't work for you, don't do it. The point is to make gradual changes until the Un-Diet is your normal way of eating.

Not eating, eating too much, or eating the wrong things backfires. The Un-Diet won't. Unlike traditional diets, it doesn't have a beginning or an end; it's simply a lifestyle—something you incorporate into your life a little at a time. You're not *on* it or *off* it as with other diets. It's not a diet; it's a way of life.

PART IV | Movement for Bouncing Back

15 | The Laws of Movement

As tired as you may be right now, and as much as you may not want to get out of that rocking chair or recliner, it is vital that you do if you want to bounce back. You can start now or delay beginning, but the sooner you start, the easier it will be.

While you were pregnant, the most obvious change to your body was the increasing size of your belly. The additional weight put pressure on your spinal cord and weakened the muscles along the front of your abdomen (the *rectus abdominis* muscles). In order for your body to accommodate this, you adjusted your posture and changed your center of gravity. Your upper body began to tilt back as your weight pulled your spine forward.

Changes that weren't so apparent, however, took place within your body. Because your body had to make room for your growing uterus and baby, it pushed many of your internal organs out of the way. You probably noticed the additional pressure on your bladder with your many frequent trips to the rest room; on your diaphragm and heart from your shortness of breath; and on your stomach and large and small intestines in your struggling digestive system.

Because God designed your body so perfectly, it isn't long after giving birth when your internal organs return to their original positions and your spinal cord readjusts to its old center of gravity. This is the beginning of your body's postbaby recovery. But you can help it along.

Your body was designed to move. In fact, in order to keep your heart, lungs, spinal cord, muscles, arteries, and other organs healthy and functioning properly, you *must* move on a continual basis. All bodies need regular participation in sustained periods of movement, but exercise will especially help *your* Body by God bounce back more quickly.

Movement doesn't require fancy equipment or tight-fitting spandex exercise outfits. God simply meant for you to be active and mobile to keep your body healthy. Historically, women accomplished that by all the walking they did. Today, because of modern technology, we walk and move less than ever before. We are a society that rides in cars, takes elevators and escalators, and sits. We sit watching television. We sit playing video games, and many of us sit at our desks or computers eight hours a day at our jobs. Because of this, we have to add movement as an essential ingredient to our daily routines, and it is not as hard as you might think.

We can easily accomplish this by inserting small *moments of movement* into every nook and cranny of our lives. You might begin by taking the stairs instead of the elevator or park in the row farthest away from the grocery store. You can take your baby for a ten-minute walk in the stroller morning and night. This is an excellent way to get a little fresh air, movement, and often lull your baby to sleep. While you're waiting for the baby bottle to heat up in the microwave, do ten deep knee bends or push-ups on the counter. You can fit movement in a lot of different places and times of the day. Any and all moments of movement assist your body in its recovery process.

Once Nicole was born, I expected to be able to slip back into my prepregnancy jeans immediately. Obviously it didn't happen. Even though I practiced moments of movement throughout my day for the first few weeks, I knew I had to step up my routine to regain my prepregnancy body. I was still physically exhausted most of the time, but I knew movement and exercise were the first steps to regaining some of my old energy.

Your resting must take place in the first few weeks, but once you get the OK from your health-care provider to begin exercising, you should add this to your schedule. Your baby will take several naps during the day. During his or her morning nap, exercise. Instead of making you more tired, this will actually give you more energy to help you get through the day. If you are tired in the afternoon, feel free to nap during your baby's afternoon nap. You'll rest better knowing that you've already exercised for the day.

Don't let the words *treadmill* or *pumping iron* scare you away, however. You do not have to go to a gym or have a stack of weights or a machine in your house. That's all fine, but movement is just that—movement. God rewards you for taking care of yourself and moving whether you do it through walking and lifting sacks of potatoes or bags of flour, or going to the gym and using the best of equipment.

The Amazing Benefits of Movement

Once you begin, there are amazing benefits of moving your Body by God through exercise.

- Exercise raises energy.
  (We all need this with a newborn.)
- It lowers blood pressure.
  (Did you know blood pressure often becomes elevated during pregnancy?)
- It reduces body fat.
  (We all can relate to this after having a baby.)
- It enhances and balances hormone production.
  (Most women are on a hormonal roller coaster during and after pregnancy.)
- It aids in the sleeping process.
  (While sleep may be a thing of the past for the next few months, it sure helps to sleep well when you can.)

- Exercise increases stress tolerance.
  (Even good stress is better when handled properly.)
- It reduces depression.
  (You are not alone if you experience postpartum depression.)
- It eliminates toxins.
- It increases bone mass.
- It decreases total and LDL cholesterol (*bad* cholesterol).
- It increases HDL cholesterol (*good* cholesterol).
- It improves heart function.
- It controls or prevents diabetes (blood sugar issues).
- It decreases the risk of injury to the muscles, joints, and spine.

The Motivation for Movement

After reviewing these benefits, you should feel a lot of motivation to fit movement into your schedule. But for many, this won't be enough. What motivates one person doesn't necessarily work for another. You have to find your own unique *motivation button*. What will trigger a big enough response from you to replace your old habits with healthier ones?

For some of you, it will be the simple fact that you want to obtain and maintain good health. You want to be there for your child as he or she grows up. You don't want untimely heart disease, diabetes, cancers, or other illnesses cutting your life short. While most women will not focus on disease, recognizing that your health is as important to your children as it is to you might help to motivate you to incorporate healthy exercise habits into your schedule. By doing so, you also set a good example for your children, helping them to realize early on the importance of taking care of their bodies. *Do what I say and not what I do* doesn't work. Your child will emulate your lifestyle and habits. For other women, looks may be their main motivation. I know many women who would never consider *not* working out for fear that they would gain weight and never regain their previous shapes and sizes. Unfortunately, some women take this motivation button (looks) to an extreme. Due to their excessive desire to stay looking *perfect*, they might try Botox injections, tummy tucks, liposuction, and other plastic surgeries. With the recent exposure extreme makeovers are getting, many feel encouraged to take dangerous and artificial routes to change their bodies.

God doesn't make mistakes. If looks are your main motivation, try doing it God's way, not the most recent television show's way.

There are numerous motivation buttons, everything from not being able to afford new clothes to envisioning someone else's unhealthy and overweight body each time you look into the mirror. Whatever it might be, it will be unique to you and a result of your upbringing, experiences, learned behavior, and habits. Something deep inside of you must be triggered in order to implement changes in your life. Unfortunately, I can't tell you exactly what that is. You will need to look deep inside of yourself and pray for the answers.

While writing this book, I did just that. It was then, for the first time in my life, that I came to grips with my past eating disorders. I had developed my habits as a result of my early experiences with weight. I would most likely be continuing those habits except that I found the motivation I needed to change them. I wanted a body that God could use for His purpose to help others. I knew that in order for this to happen, I needed a healthy body. That was my motivation button; I pray that you find yours.

After incorporating exercise into my routine, I also realized that I loved how I felt *after* exercising. After getting past those first few weeks, I started to get a good feeling. I also gained a satisfaction from pushing myself. At first it was the challenge to run around the block. When I accomplished it, it felt great. Then I was able to set another goal. This made me feel good about myself and helped me to look forward to working out. Getting started is still often the toughest part of exercising, but if I keep in mind how I feel after I am done, it gives me the motivation I need to continue working out day after day.

Use It or Lose It!

After your baby's birth, your body is at a critical juncture. It is working hard to bounce back on the inside and wants to bounce back on the outside, but it needs your help. You now have to make a choice: you can treat your Body by God with respect and use it to bounce back, or you can show it disrespect and lose it.

God has given every one of us the freedom of choice. We can choose to honor our bodies or not. Either way, because our bodies are designed to adapt to our environments, our Bodies by God *will* adapt to the choices we make in relation to them. They will adapt positively to some choices we make and will adapt negatively to others.

The law of adaptation states that over time, our Body by God will adapt to whatever environment we subject it to. My beliefs differ from Charles Darwin's, but he made the statement: "It is not the strongest of the species that survives, nor the most intelligent; it is the one that is most adaptable to change." God has created a perfect body adaptable to change.

Consider the parts of our bodies that adapt to climate, such as our skin color and temperature. Moving from Pennsylvania to Florida required my body to be able to adapt to the warmer temperatures, and my skin darkened to protect me from the abundance of ultraviolet rays.

For better or worse, your body *will* adapt, and it will adapt to your moving or your lack of it. As evident in American society's increasing waistlines and higher prevalence of heart disease and cancer, it's obvious that women's bodies are adapting and responding to their lack of movement by getting weaker, fatter, and sicker.

In contrast, if you participate in regular movement and exercise, your body will adapt and get stronger, leaner, and healthier, as God intended. So keep in mind, *you use it or lose it*. Don't feel as if it is a lost cause, however, if you did not start moving right after your child was born. You still have time to start. It is never too late to begin. Even ninety-year-old women have shown improvement in their physical health after beginning a lightweight training and exercise program (see www.seniornet.org). It's never too late to start and bounce back.

Suzie never exercised after her second child was born. She didn't lose the weight she gained during her pregnancy, and over the next few years she gained a few more pounds. Five years later, when her daughter entered kindergarten, she made a commitment to begin an exercise program. She started slowly, by walking around the block three times a week. She enjoyed looking at the houses and yards to see what was new.

Within a couple of weeks, she noticed that she was walking faster and no longer out of breath. At that time she had a routine physical and learned her cholesterol was very high. Determined to lower it without drug intervention, she continued her walking, but at a brisker rate, and she started adding one or two Foods by God at each of her meals. Thirty days later, she had her blood retested, and her cholesterol was in the normal range.

Suzie felt better than she had in a long time. Even though she hadn't dropped all the weight she hoped to, she saw she was making progress. She also noticed that she had more energy for her children when they got home from school, and that she did not become stressed as easily. Her life was changing for the good—physically and mentally—and it all started with a simple walk. Even though she began moving five years after her pregnancy, she was still able to make progress.

God Helps Mothers Who Move

Movement Gives You Energy

As I stated earlier, one of the great benefits of regular exercise and movement is the added energy it gives you. God knew that you would need all the energy you could get once you became a mother! Let's face it: even though being a mother is very rewarding, it is also very tiring. Exercise will help to keep your body at its optimum level and give you the stamina you need to help you meet your child's needs and keep up with him or her.

Movement Helps You Sleep

The added energy you gain from movement is necessary for those waking hours, but it will all come to a crashing halt without enough sleep. During the first year of motherhood, a good, sound sleep is something you only vaguely remember from the past. It's still amazing to me that a baby can wake screaming, be changed and fed, and immediately fall back into a nice, peaceful sleep. I, on the other hand, leapt from my bed startled by my baby's cries. I sleepwalked through feeding and changing her, and when I put her back to bed, I was often so exhausted or so wide awake, I *couldn't* fall back asleep.

I've mentioned that Nicole didn't sleep through the night until she was seven months old. Thankfully, after a few weeks I adopted her behavior and could fall back to sleep once she settled down as well. But even then, I didn't sleep *soundly*. I'm not sure at what age, or if at any age, a mother has the ability to sleep without still having an ear out for her child. Even though a mother may appear to be sleeping, she often wakes the second she hears a strange or abnormal gurgle, whimper, or cry from her child.

While deep, peaceful sleep may not be in the cards for a few months or even a year down the road, exercise does help you sleep better when you have the opportunity. I found that taking Nicole for a brisk walk before bedtime helped us both sleep better.

Movement Increases Your Stress Tolerance

New motherhood often brings a time of stress. The lack of sleep may contribute to this, but mothers stress over many different things, from whether or not they will be good mothers to whether the baby is eating enough or progressing in a healthy manner. Even though there is great happiness associated with having a child, every aspect and every stage brings great joy *and* stress—both good and bad.

Stress is universal, so I'm certain that all the women of the Bible had stress in some form. Even Mary most likely stressed over Jesus and her ability to mother Him. But stress on the body is not good in any form, and often with it comes increased blood pressure. Movement and exercise combine to help lower blood pressure and stress levels.

New mothers also often feel stress over their bodies. If this is the case, give yourself a break, and relax a bit. Your initial focus should be on relaxation.

Movement Helps Hormones and Depression

Do the words *hormonal roller coaster* ring any bells? The hormonal changes that a woman experiences during the nine months of pregnancy, as well as several months that follow delivery, can send any woman on an intense ride of emotional highs and lows. We've noted that these changes can often cause mood swings and sometimes feelings of depression.

Movement and exercise enhance and balance hormone production, which will help to balance your temperament and return you to your prebaby hormonal environment. They will also help to increase endorphins, your natural feel-good hormones that help to reduce depression.

Movement Helps Reduce Body Fat

As you look in the mirror hoping to see your old body but instead see a round belly and added inches on your hips and thighs, you'll probably want to cry—I did. But movement and exercise will help you reduce body fat and bounce back. This isn't simply about losing weight; it is about losing fat in the places it has accumulated during your pregnancy. The point of your movement should be to increase real muscle and decrease fat in these areas. While your main focus right now may be your appearance and how this added weight makes you look and feel, your real focus should be that this additional body fat accumulation is unhealthy. Unhealthy deposits of fat subject your body to potential problems down the road. Movement will reduce the likelihood of those problems.

 Body by God Owner's Caution—Fat vs. Muscle

Fat

- Fat has a tendency to produce more fat.
- Fatty tissue is inefficient and burns few calories.
- Fat will make you tired and lazy.
- Fat gives you a poor self-image and decreased libido.
- Fat increases your risk of nearly all disease, as well as the need for larger dress sizes and bigger pants.

Muscle

- Muscle has a tendency to produce more muscle.
- Muscle tissue works more efficiently and burns more calories.
- Muscle increases your energy.
- Muscle enhances confidence and libido.
- Increased lean muscle mass will lower your risk of certain diseases and increase your risk of looking good in clothes.

▲ ▲ ▲

Exercise by God

God didn't give Adam and Eve a treadmill, weight machines, bar-bells, and elliptical trainers to keep in shape. Man created all those pieces of exercise equipment, along with fitness gyms and workout clothing. If you walk into any gym today you will probably see fifty to one hundred different machines each for the purpose of training different muscles. You will also probably see many young women with perfect bodies in spandex outfits doing the latest aerobics or spinning exercises. Just thinking about squeezing your body into an outfit like that and exercising using man's equipment and rules can be intimidating and overwhelming.

But God didn't want you to worry about such things, so He created a perfect body that could do Exercise by God and be fit and healthy and bounce back from pregnancy.

Before the dawn of technology, everything having to do with survival required that you move. You had to build your own shelter, which required lifting, stretching, and using your muscles. You had to grow or hunt for your own food, which entailed digging and planting, and running and throwing. And the only transportation you had was your own two feet. You walked everywhere you went.

Even though things have changed dramatically since then, the same principles apply. All that God did was good. He saw that using our legs to walk and run was good. He saw that having arms to swing and lift, and muscles that could stretch and push and pull, were all good. This still stands true. Exercise by God is safe, natural, and fun, and it doesn't require expensive equipment, gym memberships, or trainers with biceps the size of your thighs. You can do everything that God has planned for helping your body to bounce back simply and in the comfort of your own home or neighborhood.

Tips for Exercising

The following tips will help to reduce or eliminate health or exercise injuries, will increase your desire to exercise, and will help you stick to your program.

Get Medical Clearance

Before beginning any exercise program, make sure that your physician has cleared you to begin. You do not want to start before your body is ready.

Wear Proper Workout Clothing

Wear loose-fitting, comfortable clothing—and sneakers and bras with good support.

Warm Up

It is critical to warm up your muscles and joints to help increase circulation before exercising. This will drastically reduce your chance of injury. Warm up for five to ten minutes before beginning your exercise session.

Stretch

Before doing any exercise, stretch for five to ten minutes to help warm up the muscles to prevent injuries.

Start Off Moderately

Keep in mind that you do not have to be Superwoman. Don't exercise to the point of exhaustion or lift so much weight that your muscles cannot move the next day, or worse, are injured. Listen to your body and do not overdo it. You have plenty of time to increase your workout.

Hydrate

Drink plenty of water before, during, and after to keep your body hydrated. A hydrated body enhances your performance; dehydration reduces performance.

Cool Down

Make sure you take five to ten minutes to help your body recover after your workout by slowing down, cooling down, and slowly stretching.

Find a Workout Partner

Having a workout partner with similar goals will help keep you on track. You can motivate and encourage each other as well as make sure that each of you is doing the exercises properly to prevent injury.

Set Fitness Goals

Without a goal, you do not know where you are going. Set realistic and specific short-term and long-term fitness goals. When you reach them, make sure you reward yourself.

Mix It Up

You don't have to do the same thing each day. Change your routines every few weeks so you don't get bored. You might walk one day, swim the next, and ride a bike another. There are lots of ways to achieve a great workout.

16 | Aerobic Exercise for Bouncing Back

Once you have the okay to begin an exercise program, the foremost question on your mind will most likely be: *How long will it take me to bounce back and get my prepregnancy body back?* There is no hard-and-fast rule on this one either. Some of my friends looked as good as they did before having a child within one month, while others took up to nine months to regain their prepregnancy sizes. A lot had to do with how much weight they had gained during pregnancy. Generally speaking, give yourself six months to a year to fully bounce back.

Just the thought of taking six to twelve months to get back into shape may depress you, but you also may be one of the lucky ones who can get back into shape very quickly. It will be easier on you mentally and physically if you set realistic goals for yourself. Your body has just been stretched to its limits—literally! Your first consideration needs to be your personal circumstances, and your second consideration should be the *gradual* reintroduction of exercise into your routine. You will need to begin slowly and tailor your workout to your own health situation.

What Is Aerobic Exercise?

Aerobic exercise, also known as *cardiovascular (cardio) exercise*, is any exercise that increases your heart rate and requires the use of oxygen. It conditions three of the most important muscles in your Body by God: your heart and two lungs.

By moving for a sustained period of at least fifteen minutes, all the organs, vessels, and glands of the cardiovascular system adapt in a healthy way. Your heart gets stronger, and your lung capacity and efficiency improve. Aerobic exercise also causes your body to process more oxygen, your body's most important nutrient. While your body could last weeks without food and days without water, you can only last a few minutes without oxygen.

You can perform cardiovascular exercise by running, walking briskly, swimming, climbing, biking, dancing, or playing a sport. You do not have to attend an aerobic dance class. The key is simply movement for a sustained period of time. While fifteen minutes is the minimum time it takes, twenty or thirty minutes may be even more beneficial.

You may be thinking, *How am I going to find a half-hour away from my baby to get out of the house?* You don't have to necessarily. With the wonderful invention of jogging strollers, you can get a great workout and your baby will enjoy the movement and fresh air. Once your child is bigger, putting her in a bicycle baby seat means biking can be fun for both of you. If these two options don't interest you, put the baby in a snuggle sling, back carrier, or stroller and take a walk. Don't forget about Daddy! Enlist the help of your spouse or a friend to swap baby-watching times so that you can get the workouts you need and deserve.

When I first made the decision to incorporate aerobic exercise into my schedule, I was a young, practicing chiropractor just out of college. My time schedule made it very difficult to get to the gym. I had run a little cross-country in high school and decided to give running a try because I felt it would be the easiest exercise to fit into my hectic schedule.

My first day out I couldn't even run a mile, but I didn't give up. Three times a week I put on my running shoes and forced myself to run again. Eventually I ran a mile, and then gradually it got easier, and I was able to run farther and farther. It wasn't long before I was running five to six miles each time. I actually began to enjoy it. I began to look forward to my runs simply because of how they made me feel.

Many women I have spoken with have expressed their frustration with aerobic exercise. They say it is difficult, and they just don't like it. My advice is to hang in there and keep doing it. You will get to the point where you break through that wall of frustration into a sense of enjoyment and well-being, as I did. It didn't happen overnight. As I said, I forced myself to run three times a week at the beginning. Now, if I don't have the opportunity to run, I actually long for it.

Aerobic exercise is anything that gets your heart pumping and your oxygen flowing. Julie wanted to begin an exercise program but didn't think running was for her because she didn't want to be too far from home at any given time. One day, while outside playing with her young children, she found herself jumping rope with them and singing "Down in the Valley." She was laughing and enjoying herself when she realized that her heart was beating fast and that jumping rope might be an excellent way to get her aerobic exercise.

Julie now jumps rope daily. She can jump in her hallway while the baby is sleeping or playing, or she can jump rope outside with her children after they get home from school. Recently I saw her jumping rope back and forth from her house to her neighbors'. She found an excellent form of aerobic exercise that met her needs perfectly.

The Potential Benefits of Aerobic Exercise

Aerobic exercise will help you bounce back more effectively and efficiently. All areas of your health will benefit.

Lungs
- Better levels of oxygen in the body
- Better absorption of oxygen by the body

- Increased lung function during exercise
- Increased lung capacity
- Increased deflation of respiratory gases, allowing the efficient removal of carbon monoxide waste from the body through the lungs

Heart

- Reduced risk of heart disease
- A stronger and larger heart, increasing the amount of oxygen-carrying blood it sends to the body with each beat
- A slower resting heart rate, because it is getting more blood to the body per beat

Blood Vessels

- Reduced blood pressure, both systolic and diastolic
- Reduced bad cholesterol
- Increased good cholesterol
- Reduced risk of hardening of the arteries
- Improved circulation
- More blood vessels form and existing ones enlarge and become more flexible
- Improved carrying capacity of the blood vessels to better carry oxygen to the body and unwanted materials away from the body

General Well-Being

- Increased fat burning and loss of weight
- Improved immune system
- Improved self-image, self-esteem, and confidence
- Reduced stress and improved ability to relax
- Improved mental alertness

Your Program for Aerobic Exercise

If you have just given birth, the past nine months were a time of decreased activity. The four weeks that followed delivery gave you an opportunity for some movement, but it was still fairly limited. Now is the time for the reintroduction of aerobic exercise.

Obviously, my passion is running and I love to be outside, even in rain or snow. This is the best option for me to get my aerobic exercise. You might find that you prefer bicycling, swimming, or an aerobics class. Aerobic exercise should not be drudgery and something you dread. You should find the activities that you most enjoy and work them into your program.

Again, you don't have to limit yourself to one form of exercise. Mix it up, and do something different each day of the week. Whatever best suits your needs is the way to go because the more you enjoy your program, the more likely you will be to stick with it.

Your program for aerobic exercise also needs to be tailored specifically to you. You can follow the guidelines beginning on the next page, describing fat burning zones, or seek the initial help of a physical trainer who will recommend what you should do based on your body size and current physical endurance. Your pace will be dependent on your individual heart rate, age, body, and fitness level.

You should not allow your heart rate to increase too much or too fast because you will tire quickly, release a lot of lactic acid into your bloodstream, create pain in your muscles and joints, increase your chance of injury, and overstress your heart. A heart monitor can help you keep an eye on your rate. You need to focus on a comfortable level of increasing your heart rate over a sustained period of at least fifteen minutes, and you may want to invest in a heart-rate monitor to help you in your initial days or months of exercise.

The safest way to start any cardiovascular exercise is by moving very slowly. If you are running, start by walking, then jogging slowly for five minutes. Whatever exercise you do, go slowly at first, then increase your speed, and then level off until you reach your moving zone. (Your moving zone is the rate at which your heart should be beating in order to get the maximum benefit from your workout. I'll show you how to calculate this in the pages ahead.) By slowly and steadily raising your heart rate, you encourage your body to burn fat right from the beginning of your workout.

The first mile is always the hardest for me, but by the second or third, my heart rate has leveled off into my perfect moving zone, and I feel as if I could run for hours. This is the point where I reach the *runner's high* that you may have heard about. It is a wonderful feeling and makes my exercise really enjoyable.

When my run is done, I make sure to cool down slowly—let my heart rate drop back to my warm-up rate. This phase helps the body slow down and redirect blood flow from the large working muscles back to the organs and brain.

Whatever your exercise, your warm-up and cool-down phase should each last five to ten minutes.

▶ Exercise Tip: It's Easier Than You Think

Even though a minimum of fifteen minutes of aerobic exercise is recommended, moving two or three times a day for ten minutes has many of the same benefits as exercising for a straight twenty or thirty minutes.

Fat Burning Zones

Your fat burning zones are the heart rates you want for experiencing exercise that is effective, pain-free, healthy, and as highly fat burning as possible. You should focus on and stay in Zones 2 and 3.

Zone #1: Maximum Heart Rate (MHR)

Your maximum heart rate is the number of beats per minute your heart should *not* exceed during exercise.

Zone #2: Fat Utilization Rate (FUR)

The fat utilization rate is a comfortable way for anyone at any level to exercise and burn fat five to seven days a week.

Zone #3: Performance Enhancement Rate (PER)

This rate enhances your athletic performance and helps you make gains in both distance and speed while still burning fat. There is also some increase in calorie output at this level without getting into sugar burning. (Fat burning is more desirable because it offers long-term benefits; sugar burning utilizes your fuel supply, or energy, which only brings short-term results.)

Zone #4: Sugar Utilization Rate (SUR)

The sugar utilization rate is at or near maximum heart rate. At this level, there is high caloric output, but also a great deal of dangerous stress being placed on your Body by God joints and cardiovascular system.

Calculating Your Moving Zone Heart Rate

Maximum Heart Rate (MHR) = 220 – Your Age
Fat Utilization Rate (FUR) = 55 to 75 percent of MHR
Performance Enhancement Rate (PER) = 75 to 85 percent of MHR

For Fat Burning Rates (FUR and PER)

- Raise by five beats if you are regularly exercising.
- Raise by ten beats if you are an experienced athlete.
- Lower by five beats if you are just starting out.
- Lower by ten beats if you are on medication or recovering from injury or illness.

Sugar Utilization Rate (SUR):

Sugar Utilization Rate = 85 to 95 percent of MHR

Your Heart Rate Zone

To find your heart rate, simply place two fingers (your forefinger and second finger) lightly but firmly over the inside of your wrist or on your neck just below the angle of your jaw. *(Caution: Do not put too much pressure on the neck; this can slow down the heart, make you dizzy, make you pass out, and can be dangerous for anyone with potential blockages of blood vessels in the neck.)* You can also place your hand over your heart to count the number of beats, or if you prefer, simply use a heart-rate monitor.

Once you find your heartbeat, count your heartbeats (pulse) for ten seconds with a watch, then multiply this number by six to get your heartbeats per minute. Determine your target heart rate and check your pulse every five minutes to make sure that you are staying within your desired heart range. If not, increase or decrease your level of activity to get back into the zone that you desire.

Running Posture and Position

- Head and shoulders back.
- Back straight.
- Eyes facing straight ahead.
- Arms stay bent at your sides.
- Breathe in through your nose and fill your stomach with air right behind your belly button. Breathe out slowly through your mouth by contracting your chest.

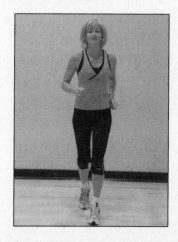

- Gently roll your feet from heel to toe.
- Don't work any harder than you have to, or work as hard as you can. It all depends on your goal.

Choose Your Rate Based on Your Goal

Goal #1: Fat Utilization Rate (FUR)

Movement is at a comfortable, steady pace you enjoy. FUR moves you into a moderate, aerobic, fat burning state, which will safely help you lose fat and increase your overall health.

Goal #2: Performance Enhancement Rate (PER)

Movement is at a swifter rate of speed that is sustainable. PER helps you increase your efficiency and learn to be more productive as you move. This rate will continue to burn fat for fuel while increasing performance times and efficiency. PER is used in preparation for performing in events that require sustained movement, such as long-distance running.

Goal #3: Sugar Utilization Rate (SUR)

Movement is up-tempo, challenging, and there is a limit to how long you can sustain the exercise. SUR provides your body with the ability to perform at high intensity. Athletes who participate in sports that require quick bursts of movement will benefit from training in the SUR zone. SUR training will increase performance in all activities as it enhances different components of energy output and heart, lung, and muscle function.

Goal #4: Combining FUR, PER, and SUR

To increase your heart rate and move from FUR to PER to SUR, you can perform the movement faster, at a steeper incline, or increase the weight or tension, depending on the form of exercise.

Sample Aerobic Routines

To set up your own personal aerobic program:

1. Calculate your moving zones.
2. Choose an exercise.
3. Begin the exercise with a five- to ten-minute warm-up.
4. Move through the exercise, increasing the speed, tension, or incline so you can achieve or stay in the right zone.
5. Finish the exercise with a five- to ten-minute cooldown.
6. Following the activity, write down what speed, tension, or incline was necessary to achieve the particular zone.

Don't Forget to Drink

Whether you sweat a lot or not, keeping your body hydrated while you are working out is critical. When your heart rate goes up, the water levels in your body go down. This can cause strain on your heart, and your joints will get dry, making them painful and susceptible to injury. You may also feel symptoms similar to those of low blood sugar. You may feel light-headed, dizzy, or nauseous.

Whenever a friend of mine went for her morning runs, she always stopped short because she felt light-headed. She attributed it to her low blood sugar. She continued to run but kept a box of raisins or other fruit with her at all times so that when she began to feel sick, she could raise her blood sugar immediately. But this didn't help either, and she was about to give up her exercise completely when I suggested she drink more fluids. She tried it, and she no longer had any symptoms. Symptoms of dehydration will often mimic those of hypoglycemia.

A good rule of thumb is to drink one liter of water per hour of aerobic exercise. Again, drink before, during, and after exercising. If you are exercising anywhere other than in your home, take a water bottle with you in your hand, on a belt, or in a backpack that is easily accessible.

It's a good idea to drink water constantly throughout the day. A general rule is that you need one-half your body weight in ounces of water every day. So if you weigh 128 pounds, you would need to drink sixty-four ounces (two quarts) of water daily whether you are exercising or not.

 Oh, No! Not Again!

If you think one infant is a lot of work, try adding eleven other children of various ages. One thing is for certain: there is precious little downtime for Mom! Just imagine half a dozen toddlers all careening around the yard on tricycles and scooters. Then add three or four tweenies shooting hoops. Then throw in several teenagers walking around with CD players attached to their ears, oblivious to everything else. If you don't think a mother in this situation has to keep moving, you are about to be proven wrong!

The physicality of bringing a child into the world doesn't end with the birth. Every child requires a parent to keep up with him or her (literally), so after your baby is born, you will be moving a lot. Rachel and Leah were both married to Jacob, the patriarch of the nation of Israel. These two women and their maids were responsible for no fewer than twelve children and their welfare. Rachel and Leah, Bilhah and Zilpah were definitely women on the move!

With all those babies being born, the women's bodies didn't have a lot of time for bouncing back from the stresses (and stretches) of pregnancy. And with all those children running around, there wasn't a lot of time for going to the gym to get back into shape. However, their entire lives were about exercise—simply due to having to keep up with and care for all the children! If this weren't the case, they probably would not have been healthy enough to go on, but God helped them fit in their aerobic exercise even though they may not have realized they were doing it.

—Scripture reference: Genesis 29:1–30:24

▲ ▲ ▲

17 | You Must Resist for Bouncing Back

Resistance training increases your muscle mass. Muscle burns more calories than fat, which ultimately helps you toward your goal of bouncing back. Muscle mass is necessary for keeping your Body by God healthy. It is also going to be a major factor over the next few months as your child grows.

If you are wondering why, try carrying around a five-pound bag of sugar in one arm for an hour straight. If you don't think you will ever hold your baby this much, you are in for a surprise! Then, as an experiment, take a ten-pound bag of flour and try to hold that for even thirty minutes. You will find that the muscles in your arms and back will tire very quickly without strong and healthy muscle support. It is important that you build up your strength and muscles slowly and properly to avoid injury.

I don't want you to begin to panic and think I expect you to become a bodybuilder with bulging muscles. No, you will not look like Arnold Schwarzenegger or Sylvester Stallone. That's not the plan. I lift weights two to three times a week, and as you can see from my photo, I do not look like a muscle man with breasts! Resistance training is simply good for you and will aid in your bouncing back more quickly. It will also give you the nice, fit look, especially in your upper body, that you desire and need.

Personally, I never liked lifting weights. I would have chosen running twelve miles, biking for twenty, or swimming lap after lap over lifting any day of the year. Unfortunately, no matter how much I ran, biked, or swam, I couldn't get rid of my baby belly. I had lost the weight I had gained during pregnancy. In fact, I was thinner and weighed less than I had before getting pregnant, yet I still had fat on my stomach that wouldn't go away. I could have run a marathon daily, and I'm certain that baby belly would have bounced along with me day after day.

I asked every woman I knew what to do about this. Finally, my husband, Ben, suggested lifting weights and doing resistance training. He figured it couldn't hurt, and might help. I began doing some weight training and resistance exercises, and my belly went away. I was sold and it was all the motivation I needed! I incorporated these exercises into my routine two times a week for twenty minutes each time. While some days this twenty minutes feels like a chore, I remind myself of the results I saw, and continue to see, as a benefit for taking this time.

In fact, I now have an added benefit to my lifting weights. All of my life I have had trouble with a condition that makes me hunch over. This has caused me backaches since I can remember. I lived with this pain for close to thirty years, but when I began doing resistance training, the pain went away. I know resistance training will always be part of my training program due to the overwhelmingly positive effects it has had on my life.

The Potential Benefits of Resistance Training

Resistance training is also known as *weight* or *strength training*. It is important to incorporate this type of exercise into your routine in order for your body to bounce back more effectively and efficiently. Here are other added benefits of resistance training.

- It increases your ability to perform daily activities.
- It increases your strength.

- It increases your muscle tone.
- It increases your flexibility and coordination.
- It increases your lean muscle tissue.
- It boosts your self-esteem and image.
- It reduces your blood pressure and cholesterol.
- It provides an outlet from postbaby stress.
- It helps you eliminate the baby fat deposited around your midsection.

The Terminology of Resistance Movement

Before we begin, let me explain: resistance exercise is applying sustained or repetitive strain (resistance) to your muscle. The most effective way to create this resistance against your muscles and produce the best results is a properly applied weight-lifting program.

Resistance weight training also has its own unique vocabulary. You will need to be familiar with these terms and have a proper understanding of the weight resistance program to start. We'll begin with some definitions.

Repetitions (or Reps)

A repetition is how many times you do the specified exercise. If you lift a weight twelve times, that is twelve repetitions, or reps.

Sets

A set is a group of repetitions or how many separate times you perform the repetitions of the exercise. For instance, three sets of twelve repetitions is performing twelve repetitions, three separate times.

Failure

Doing an exercise until "failure" means performing a set until you literally cannot perform even one more rep.

Rest Periods

A rest period is the amount of rest between each set.

Intensity

Intensity refers to how challenging an exercise is. You don't have to use heavy weights or perform workouts that are unsafe or painful to get intense exercise. While adding heavier weights to your sets will increase intensity, too much weight can cause pain and injury. The safest way to increase intensity of a workout is to shorten the time between sets, or the time between each exercise. In this way, intensity not only makes your workouts more effective, it makes them more time-efficient as well.

How to Stand: Perfect Posture Equals Perfect Technique

As we discussed previously, your posture changed during pregnancy. Your body tilted back as your weight pulled you forward, muscles weakened, and pressure was put on your spinal cord. In order to bounce back more quickly, it is critical that you regain your prior perfect posture. To maximize your results and avoid possible injury, it is also critical that you use as perfect a posture as possible when doing any exercise and stretching.

God designed the body using all the vast, highly technical laws of science, mathematics, and physics in order for your Body by God to best deal with gravity. When maintaining your posture, the muscles, joints, and bones are at their strongest and most stable. This will allow them to be able to withstand forces without suffering injury.

Perfect Posture

- (A) The head is up and back so the ears line up over the shoulders, and the arc (lordosis or C curve) in the neck is maintained.

- (B) Shoulders are rolled back in the joints.
- (C) Upper back is flat and not arched or humped.
- (D) Belly button is out and hips back so you have an arc (lordosis/C curve like the neck) in your lower back, called the *weight-lifter's arch*.
- (E) Knees are slightly bent to provide shock absorption.

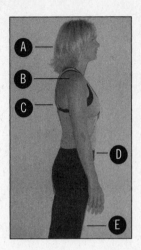

You should maintain this posture during all stretches and exercises. Any exercise that calls for a disruption of posture is unhealthy, or you are doing it wrong.

How to Stretch

Due to the changes your body went through during the nine months of your pregnancy, certain muscles weakened and got too short or too tight. Jumping into an exercise program without stretching could cause injury, pain, or degeneration over time. It is critical that you incorporate proper stretching before, during, and after any exercising or workout.

Following are some short muscles and their stretches.

Hamstrings
- (A) While sitting on the floor with your right leg straight and with your toes pointing up, bend your left leg inward so the bottom of the left foot touches the right knee.
- (B) Bend forward at the hip, bringing your chest towards your thigh. Repeat on the opposite side. (See next page.)

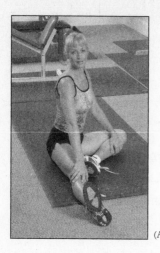 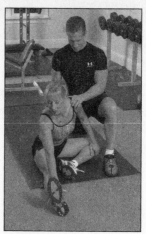

(A) (B)

Calves

Place one foot in front of the other, lean forward, placing your hands on a bench. Keep your heel close to the ground, stretching your calf. Repeat on the opposite side.

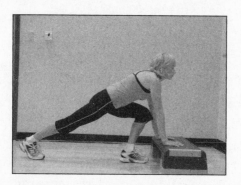

Chest Muscles / Front Shoulders

Stand by a wall or in a doorway and put your hand against it at eye level. Lean back from your hand until your arm is straight and being pulled back enough to cause a stretch in the chest and shoulder muscles. Change the level of your hand to below the waist and above your head in order to perform this stretch at three different angles.

Front of Neck

Roll your shoulders back, pull your chin in, and then roll your head back so you are looking up at the ceiling behind you. This stretches the front of your neck. The muscles and ligaments in the front of the neck get tight due to the forward head posture created by driving, watching television, or sitting at a desk or computer.

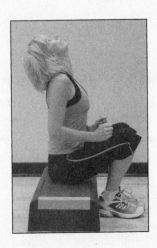

You should hold all stretches for ten to fifteen seconds, back off slightly, take a deep breath in, then let it out while you repeat the stretch for another ten to fifteen seconds. Each time you go back down while breathing out, you should be able to stretch farther. Do each stretch at least three times to achieve the maximum benefit.

How to Breathe and Count While Lifting

You may recall the shortness of breath you had while pregnant because your lungs were being pushed up and compressed to accommodate your growing baby. You knew, however, how important proper oxygen flow was to you and your baby. It is just as important in exercise to achieve proper oxygen flow to your muscles and tissues.

You do not want to hold your breath while lifting. Instead you will want to inhale or breathe in on the eccentric contraction (while you are lowering or releasing the weight), and exhale or breathe out on the concentric contraction (while you are lifting the weight).

Count one, two on the concentric contraction (when lifting). Count one, two, three, four on the eccentric contraction (when releasing or lowering the weight).

What to Lift

Free Weights

Free weights are weights that are not connected to anything. They can range in weight from one to five pounds, and then typically increase in five-pound increments. They include dumbbells, barbells, and hand and ankle weights. If you have never done any lifting, you may want to begin with five-pound weights.

Stationary Weights

Stationary weights are connected to a machine that allows various types of resistance lifts. Most gyms have a variety of stationary equipment that works different muscles. You can also find good home equipment that works various muscles depending on how the machine is set up.

Body Weight

You can use your own body weight to create resistance. An example of this is a push-up. Exercises of this type will not require any special equipment.

Remember *Use It or Lose It?*

Resistance training is not simply for you to use to get back into shape and then stop. It should become part of your lifelong exercise routine. Within forty-eight hours after performing resistance exercise, your muscles begin to atrophy. When muscles atrophy, that means they get smaller and weaker, or in other words, go away. Think how much your muscles have atrophied over the past nine months. You obviously have some work to do, so remember the law of *Use It or Lose It* and make resistance training a required part of your exercise routine. Keep in mind: no resistance means no muscles.

▲ ▲ ▲

18 | Resistance Exercises

Your abdominal area will most likely be your main focus at this point in time. Your abdomen connects your sternum to your pelvis. Therefore, the only movements that work your abs are ones that lift your sternum up while the pelvis is stabilized or ones that lift the pelvis up while the sternum is stabilized. Any movement or equipment that does neither, or more than these two movements, will not help your stomach. When it comes to abs, simplicity is best.

Abdominals

(*Denotes Preferred Exercise by God)

*Floor Crunch

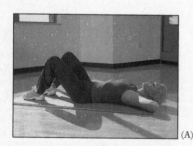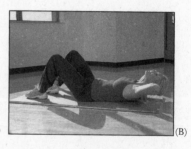

(A)   (B)

(A) Position: Lie flat on your back with your feet flat on the floor. Make a triangle out of your hands by touching your thumbs and

index fingers together, and rest your head in the center so your neck is straight and you are looking straight up toward the ceiling.

(B) Movement: Without bending your head or using your arms in any way, lift your head and sternum only a few inches up toward the ceiling—use only your stomach muscles. Pretend that an arrow is driving your belly button into the floor while at the same time a string is lifting your nose toward the ceiling. At the top of the movement, crunch your abs together for a two-count and then lower yourself down. Do not relax your abdominals at the bottom of the move. When you reach the bottom, hover slightly over the ground and then repeat the movement.

Breathe out one, two as you lift your sternum. You should be completely out of air as you crunch your abs together for a count of two. Breathe in one, two, three, four as you lower yourself back toward the floor.

Tip: Hold a weight behind your head as your abdominals get stronger. Remember to still keep your head straight.

Caution: Never hook your legs under anything when doing abdominal routines. That makes you stop using your stomach and start using your back.

*Oblique Crunch

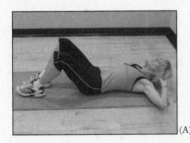 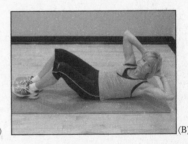

(A) (B)

(A) Position: Lie flat on your back with your feet flat on the floor. Make a triangle out of your hands and rest your head in the center so your neck is straight and you are looking straight up toward the ceiling.

(B) Movement: Lift your head up toward the ceiling as in a regular crunch, but at the top of the movement bring your elbow toward your opposite knee. Repeat for the required number of reps, and then switch to the opposite elbow and knee.

Breathe out one, two as you lift your sternum and elbow up and across. You should be completely out of air as you crunch your abs together for a two-count. Breathe in one, two, three, four as you lower yourself back toward the floor.

*Bent-Knee Leg Raise

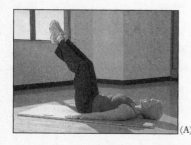 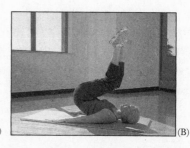

(A)   (B)

(A) Position: Lie flat on your back with your hands at your sides, palms down and your legs bent so your thighs are at a ninety-degree angle with your stomach, your knees are bent slightly toward your chest, and your feet are in the air. This can also be done on a bench with hands grabbing the top of the bench.

(B) Movement: Using your abs, lift your pelvis up off the floor toward your nose, then lower back slowly to the starting position.

Breathe out one, two as you lift your pelvis. Breathe in one, two, three, four as you lower your pelvis back down toward the floor.

Caution: This is not a leg lift. A leg lift uses your lower back. Make sure to keep your legs bent and focus on using your stomach muscles, which are responsible for lifting your pelvis off the ground.

*Side Crunch

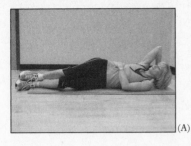 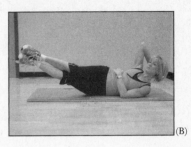

(A) (B)

(A) Position: Lie on your side with both legs slightly bent and on top of each other, and your top hand reaching down behind your head in order to hold it up.

(B) Movement: Using your side muscles, lift your head and bottom shoulder up off the ground while simultaneously lifting your feet. At the top of the movement, crunch your side muscles together for a count of two before lowering back down. When you are finished with the required number of reps, roll over and do the other side.

Breathe out one, two as you lift your head, shoulder, and feet off the floor. You should be completely out of air as you crunch your side abs together for a two-count. Breathe in one, two, three, four as you lower yourself back toward the floor.

*Side Raise

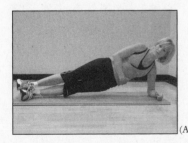 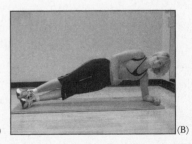

(A) (B)

(A) Position: Lie on your side on top of your elbow, with your top hand palm down on the floor and your bottom hand placed

palm down on the floor or on your hip to increase the difficulty.

(B) Movement: Lift your hip up off the ground as far as you can, hold for a count of two, and then lower. Repeat the required number of reps, then switch to the other side.

Breathe out one, two as you lift your hips off the floor. Breathe in one, two, three, four as you lower your hips back down.

Tip: You can place your top hand on your hip to make the movement more challenging.

The Lower Body

(*Denotes Preferred Exercise by God)

Lower-body resistance movements should address six main areas for women:

1. Quadriceps (the muscles on the front of the upper leg)
2. Hamstrings (the muscles on the back of the upper leg)
3. Calves (the muscles on the back of the lower leg)
4. Gluteus muscles (the muscles you sit on)
5. Inner thigh muscles (the inside of the upper leg)
6. Outer thigh muscles (the outside of the upper leg)

Squats and lunges are the most effective way to build lean muscle and strength in the body's largest and most significant areas: quadriceps, gluteus, hamstrings, and inner/outer thighs.

*One-Legged Squat (Quadriceps, Hamstrings, Glutes)

I like the one-legged squat because it is a natural movement and creates very little pressure in the shoulders and lower back. This exercise takes the hips and knees through a more natural range of motion. (See next page.)

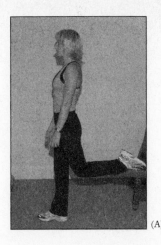
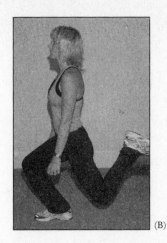

(A)   (B)

(A) Position: Find a surface (bench or chair) that is approximately knee height. Stand, in perfect posture, in front of the surface and place one foot on top of it, keeping the bench or chair behind you.

(B) Movement: Squat down with your other leg until the back of it is parallel to the floor and at an approximate ninety-degree angle to your lower leg and calf. Then stand back up to the starting position. Repeat the required number of reps, then switch to the other leg.

Breathe in one, two, three, four on the way down, and breathe out one, two on the way up.

Tip: To elevate the difficulty or intensity level, you can perform this exercise while holding weights in your hands and increasing the weight as you get stronger.

Standard (Two-Legged) Squat

This exercise is a more unnatural movement that puts a tremendous amount of pressure on the shoulders, lower back, and knees. If you are having trouble with any of these areas, avoid this squat. It is the easiest exercise by which to sustain an injury if done incorrectly. (See next page.)

(A) Position: Stand with your feet slightly more than shoulder width apart, in perfect posture, holding a dumbell in each hand.

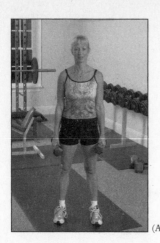 (A) 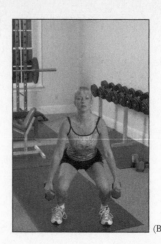 (B)

(B) Movement: Maintaining perfect posture and looking up, squat down as if getting ready to sit until the back of your legs are parallel to the floor and at a ninety-degree angle to your calves. Your lower legs and calves must remain close to perpendicular to the floor, with your knees remaining directly above your ankles and not out in front of your toes. Then stand back up to the starting position.

Breathe in one, two, three, four on the way down, and breathe out one, two on the way up.

Caution: When performing a one- or two-legged squat, do not let your knee or knees get out in front of your toes or bend over and lose perfect posture. If you feel any pain or pulling sensation in your back, knees, or hips, stop the exercise immediately and consult a health professional.

*Lunges (Quadriceps, Hamstrings, Glutes)

A lunge is another excellent safe and natural movement for working the legs, glutes, hips, and thighs. (See next page.)

(A) Position: Stand in good posture with or without weights in your hands, depending on strength and experience.

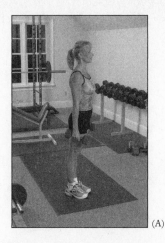
(A)

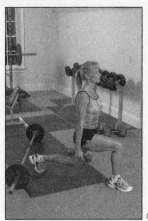
(B)

(B) Movement: Take a long step forward, bringing your center line (your groin) toward the back of your front ankle and bending your front knee until that upper leg is at a ninety-degree angle to the lower leg. The front lower leg must remain close to perpendicular to the floor, with your knee over your foot and ankle but not over your toes. Your back knee should bend down until it is two or three inches above the floor and your back toes are bent. Hold that position for a moment. Then push back with your front foot so you are back to the starting position. Repeat ten to fifteen times on that leg, and then switch legs.

Breathe in one, two, three, four on the way down, and breathe out one, two on the way up.

Caution: Do not allow your back knee to hit the ground or your front knee to extend over your toes.

Tip: To make the move more challenging, after completing the lunge, instead of pushing with your front foot back into a standing position, bring your back foot forward as if you were walking. Then step out again, always bringing your back foot up so you end up walking across the floor.

Additional Tip: A lunge is slightly easier on the knees than a one-legged squat, so it is a good exercise for those with knee problems.

Leg Extension (Quadriceps)

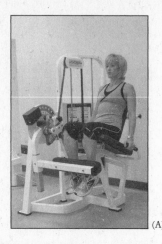 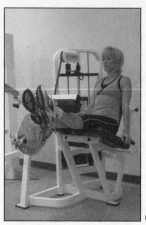

(A)   (B)

This is not an Exercise by God because it isolates one muscle group rather than being a natural movement that recruits several. Leg extensions are still great exercises because they strengthen the muscles surrounding the knee that typically become weak due to the modern lifestyle of sitting too much.

(A) Position: Sit on a leg extension machine and slide your legs under the roller pads. Hook your ankles underneath the pads so the pads are resting on top of your lower shin areas. Grab the handles or the sides of the bench.

(B) Movement: With your toes pointed out, lift your legs until your knees are straight. Hold this for a second while squeezing your quadriceps (thigh muscles), and then lower the weight slowly back to the starting position.

Breathe out one, two on the way up, and breathe in one, two, three, four on the way down.

Caution: Sit in good posture, and do not lift your bottom off the seat.

Tip: If you do not have access to a leg extension machine, you can do this at home using a paint can filled with sand. Sit in a chair and hook your foot under the handle and perform the exercise one leg at a time.

Leg Curl (Hamstrings)

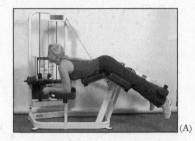
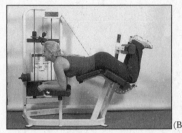

(A)　(B)

(A) Position: Lie facedown on a leg-curl machine and put your ankles under the roller pad so it is resting on the backs of your lower ankles. Keep your head arched up slightly and grab the handles or the sides of the bench you are lying on.

(B) Movement: Bend your legs until the roller pad hits the top of your hamstrings (the backs of your legs). Hold the position for a second while squeezing your hamstrings, and then slowly lower the weight back down to the starting position.

Breathe out one, two on the way up, and breathe in one, two, three, four on the way down.

Dumbbell Hamstring Curl

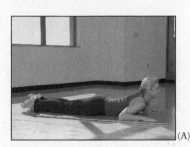
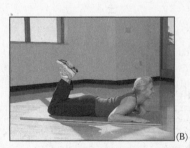

(A)　(B)

If you do not have access to a hamstring-curl machine, this can be done lying facedown on the floor. Hold a dumbbell between your feet and slowly bend your legs at the knee and raise them. Repeatedly raise and lower your legs. This can also be done on a bench with a partner placing dumbbells on and removing dumbbells from your feet.

Caution: Do not allow your hips to rise up off the bench or floor.

Dumbbell Straight-Leg Dead Lifts (Hamstrings and Lower Back)

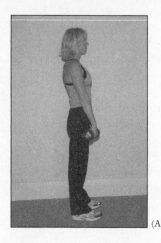 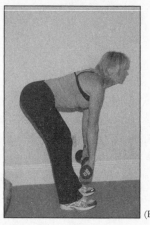

(A)   (B)

(A) Position: Stand, holding one dumbbell in each hand, with your knees a little more than slightly bent, your palms facing your legs, and an intense focus on your posture (particularly your weight-lifter's arch).

(B) Movement: Maintaining correct posture in your lower back, shoulders, and neck, lower the weights toward the floor. Stop before the weights touch the ground and/or before you feel that you must begin to lose your weight-lifter's arch, arch or hump your upper back, or drop your head and shoulders forward. Once you get to this point, reverse the movement, standing back up to the starting position. During this movement, you should feel a good stretch in your hamstrings, particularly where they tie into your gluteus muscles.

Breathe out one, two on the way up, and breathe in one, two, three, four on the way down.

Tip: This exercise can be done with a barbell. However, the barbell makes it more difficult to maintain good posture and protect your lower back.

Caution: This exercise is safe for the lower back only when done properly. Make sure to maintain good posture throughout this exercise. Again, keep the weight-lifter's arch in your lower back, do not arch or hump your upper back, and do not drop your head forward.

Abduction (Outer Thigh)

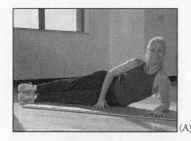 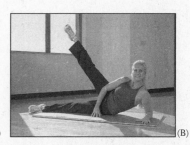

(A)   (B)

(A) Position: Lie on your side, with your knees slightly bent and your legs lying on top of each other.

(B) Movement: Lift your top leg straight toward the ceiling as high as you can, using your outer thigh and hip muscles. Hold the position for one second, and then slowly lower back down to the starting position. Repeat required number of reps, then switch sides.

Breathe out one, two on the way up, and breathe in one, two, three, four on the way down.

Adduction (Inner Thigh)

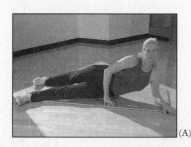 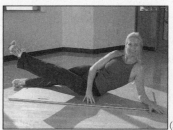

(A)   (B)

(A) Position: Lie on your side, with your bottom leg placed straight out in front of your upper leg.

(B) Movement: Lift the bottom leg, using your inner thigh and hip muscles. Hold the position for one second, then lower slowly. Repeat required number of reps, then switch sides.

Breathe out one, two on the way up, and breathe in one, two, three, four on the way down.

Tip: To make abduction and adduction more challenging, wear an ankle weight.

Additional Tip: Abduction/adduction can be performed on a machine.

*One-Legged Calf Raise (Calves)

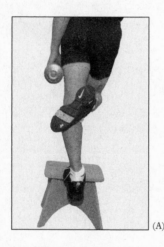 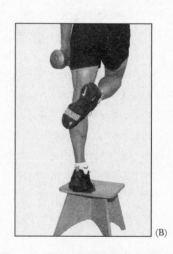

(A)   (B)

(A) Position: Start by standing with the ball of your left foot on a surface that is several inches off the ground. Hold a dumbbell (or no weight for beginners) in your left hand, and hold on to something else with your right hand to give you balance.

(B) Movement: Lower your left heel slowly toward the ground as far as possible and then lift up toward the ceiling as far as possible. When you get to the top of the movement, squeeze your calf muscle for one

second, and then slowly lower your heel back to the bottom. Repeat required number of reps, then switch to the other foot and hand.

Breathe out one, two on the way up, and breathe in one, two, three, four on the way down.

Seated Calf Raise (Calves)

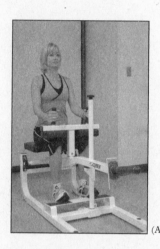 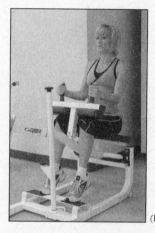

(A) (B)

(A) Position: Sit down in perfect posture on a seated calf-raise machine so the balls of your feet are on the foot platform and your knees are underneath the pads.

(B) Movement: Slowly lower your heels as far as you can and then lift the weight up as high as possible. Then slowly lower your heels all the way back to the bottom again.

Breathe out one, two on the way up, and breathe in one, two, three, four on the way down.

Tip: A seated calf raise does not work the entire calf muscle. A standing calf-raise machine or one-legged calf raise can be used to better reach the whole calf muscle.

Caution: Do not allow your ankle or knees to roll out as you lift up during any calf movement.

▶ Additional Tip: Exercise Alternative

If you do not have access to a calf machine, you can achieve a similar effect by standing on a book or on a step and lifting yourself up and down using your calf muscles.

The Upper Body

(*Denotes Preferred Exercise by God)

Upper-body resistance movements need to concentrate on the following six areas:

1. The chest
2. The triceps (the muscles on the backside of the upper arm)
3. The biceps (the muscles on the front side of the upper arm)
4. The shoulders (deltoids and rear deltoids)
5. The back (lats)
6. The abdominals

Bench presses are a good way to hit several muscle groups at one time. They work the chest, shoulders, and triceps all at once. I prefer dumbbells because they allow more natural freedom of movement than barbells do. This makes them safer, more effective, and great for Exercise by God. On the following pages you will find several more helpful Exercises by God.

Incline Dumbbell Flye Press (Chest, Shoulders, Triceps)

(A) Position: Holding two dumbbells, lie back on a bench that is at a slight incline (approximately twenty to forty degrees). Hold the weights so your palms are facing toward you and your elbows are bent so your hands are just above your body. (See next page.)

(B) Movement: Push the weights straight up over the sternum/chin

area while rotating your hands so your palms begin to face away from you and your thumbs are facing each other. Push the weights all the way up until just before your elbows are locked. Touch the weights together slightly and hold that position for one second. Then slowly lower the weight while rotating your hands so your palms are again facing you and you are back in the starting position.

Breathe out one, two on the way up, and breathe in one, two, three, four on the way down.

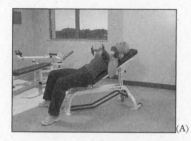 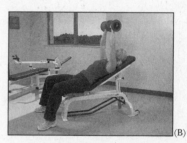

Flat Dumbbell Flye Press (Chest, Shoulders, Triceps)

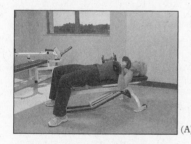 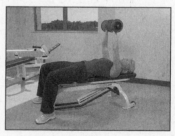

(A) Position: Holding two dumbbells, lie back on a flat bench. As with the incline flye press, hold the weights so your palms are facing toward you and your elbows are bent so your hands are just above your body.

(B) Movement: Push the weights straight up over the sternum/chin area while rotating your hands so your palms begin to face away from you and your thumbs are facing each other. Push the weights all the way up until just before your elbows are locked. Touch the weights together and hold that position for a second. Then slowly lower the

weights while rotating your hands so your palms are again facing you and you are back in the starting position.

Breathe out one, two on the way up, and breathe in one, two, three, four on the way down.

Tip: By internally rotating the hands on the way up (bringing your thumbs toward each other), you get more use out of the chest muscles.

Caution: Do not lift your head off the bench while you are lifting.

Incline Flyes (Chest)

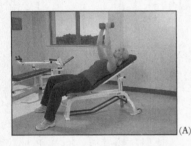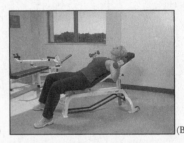

(A) (B)

(A) Position: Hold a dumbbell in each hand and lie down on a bench that is placed at a slight incline. Hold the dumbbells up over your body with your palms facing each other and your elbows slightly bent.

(B) Movement: Slowly lower the weight down and out in an arc-like movement so the weights are coming down away from your body. Lower your elbows until they are even with the bench. Hold for a count of two and then return to the top, maintaining the same arc-like path you made on the way down. At the top of the movement, squeeze.

Breathe out one, two on the way up, and breathe in one, two, three, four on the way down.

Tip: Do not let your elbows drop down below the bench or allow your arms to go out straight at the bottom of the movement.

*Incline or Flat Push-Up (Chest, Shoulders, Triceps)

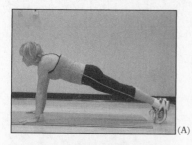
(A)

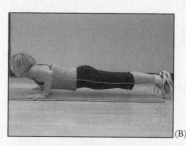
(B)

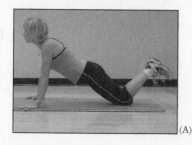
(A)

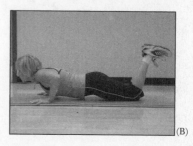
(B)

(A & B) Position and Movement: With your feet on the floor or up on a raised surface, perform push-ups, keeping your head up and your back straight.

Breathe out one, two on the way up, and breathe in one, two, three, four on the way down.

Tip: To make this movement easier, you can do the push-ups from your knees.

Caution: Do not let your hips sag down below your body or lift up above your body.

*Barbell Curl (Biceps)

(A) Position: Stand in correct posture, holding a barbell with your hands just slightly more than shoulder width apart. (See next page.)

(B) Movement: Maintain perfect posture, keeping your elbows at your sides, and curl the weight up. At the top of the movement,

squeeze your biceps for a count of two, and then slowly lower the weight back to the starting position.

Breathe out one, two on the way up, and breathe in one, two, three, four on the way down.

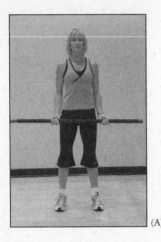 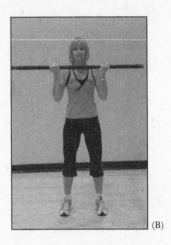

(A)   (B)

*Dumbbell Curl (Biceps)

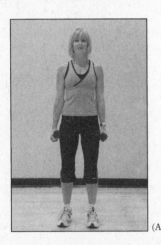 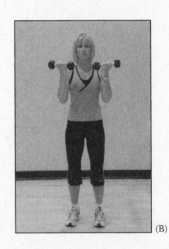

(A)   (B)

(A) Position: Stand in good posture, holding a dumbbell in each hand with your palms facing toward you.

(B) Movement: Using one arm, curl the weight while rotating your palm and thumb out away from your body. At the top of the movement, squeeze your biceps for a count of two, and then lower the weight while rotating your palm back down into the starting position. Repeat the movement using the other arm.

Breathe out one, two on the way up, and breathe in one, two, three, four on the way down.

Tip: By rotating your hands, you get more use out of the bicep muscles.

Hammer Curl (Biceps)

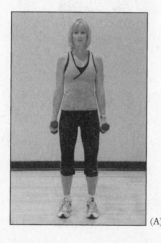 (A)   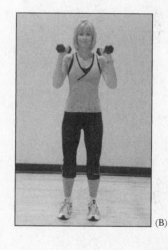 (B)

(A) Position: Stand in good posture, holding a dumbbell in each hand with your palms facing toward you.

(B) Movement: Using one arm, curl the weight up while keeping your palm facing your body. At the top of the movement, squeeze your biceps for a count of two, and then lower the weight back down into the starting position. Repeat the movement using the other arm.

Breathe out one, two on the way up, and breathe in one, two, three, four on the way down.

Tip: Do not lean far back or use momentum by swaying to lift the weight. Also, do not dig your elbows into your rib case for leverage.

*Tricep Pushdown—Rope or Bar (Triceps)

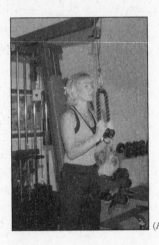

(A)

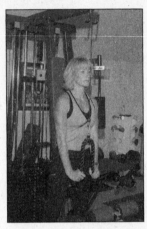

(B)

I like to use a rope if available for this movement in order to get a fuller range of motion out of the triceps. If a rope is not available, a slightly bent bar can be used to get almost the same effect.

(A) Position: Using a cable machine, grab the rope or bar with your palms facing down. The cable must be high enough so your hands are at shoulder level. Keeping the proper straight arch in your back, bend forward very slightly and pull your hands down just below shoulder level, making sure to keep your wrists straight.

(B) Movement: Push the rope or bar down toward your legs, using only your triceps and without moving the rest of your body. Push down until you completely lock your elbows. If you are using a rope, extend your hands out past your legs. At the bottom of the movement, squeeze your triceps for a count of two before slowly raising the rope or bar back up the starting position.

Breathe out one, two on the way up, and breathe in one, two, three, four on the way down.

Caution: Do not bend over and recruit your shoulders or chest to get the weight down.

One-Arm Standing Triceps Extension (Triceps)

(A) Position: Stand, holding one dumbbell straight up over your head with your palm angled slightly in toward your head and your elbow angled slightly out.

(B) Movement: Lower the weight slowly behind your head, keeping your elbow angled slightly out so you do not have to bend your head forward out of posture to get the weight behind it. Lower the weight down as far as you can, then lift it back up to the starting position. When you are back up to the top, squeeze your triceps for a count of two before performing the movement again.

Breathe out one, two on the way up, and breathe in one, two, three, four on the way down.

Caution: Do not bend your head down on this or any movement. This can cause neck strain or injury.

*One-Arm Bent Triceps Extension (Triceps)

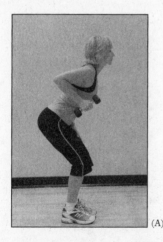
(A)
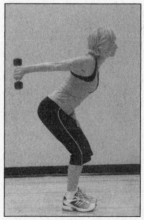
(B)

(A) Position: Stand, holding one dumbbell with your palm facing your body and then bend at the waist, keeping good posture and your back straight and your head up. Place your other hand on your knee or another surface for balance. With the arm holding the dumbbell, lift your elbow straight up and back until your upper arm (bicep/tricep) is parallel to the floor and your elbow is bent at a ninety-degree angle.

(B) Movement: Using your triceps, extend the weight back behind you until your elbow is locked out and your entire arm is parallel with the floor. At the top of the lift, squeeze your triceps for a count of two before lowering the weight back down to the starting position.

Breathe out one, two on the way up, and breathe in one, two, three, four on the way down.

Tip: You can also do this by placing your knee on a bench on the same side as the hand holding the weight and placing the other hand down at the end of the bench.

Caution: Do not swing the weight or use momentum from your body to lift it up.

Reverse Bench Dip (Triceps)

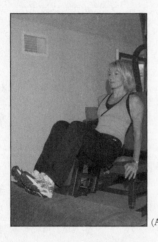
(A)

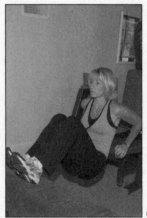
(B)

(A) Position: Place two benches or chairs approximately half a body length apart. Sit on one bench or chair while facing the other. Place your palms on the bench or chair you are sitting on while putting your feet on the other with your knees slightly bent. Then slide your bottom off of the surface you are sitting on and, using your triceps, lift yourself up by locking your arms.

(B) Movement: Lower your bottom down toward the floor until your upper arm is parallel to the floor. Then straighten your arms back out to return to the beginning position.

Breathe in one, two, three, four on the way down, and breathe out one, two on the way up.

Tip: You can have someone apply pressure to your shoulders to make the move challenging.

Caution: Do not lower yourself more than six inches from the seat of the chair.

*Triangle Push-Up (Triceps)

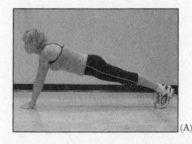 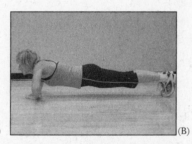

(A)   (B)

(A) Position: Make a triangle out of your hands by putting your thumbs and index fingers together.

(B) Movement: Do push-ups from the floor, with your feet up on a bench, or from your knees, if you are a beginner, by lowering your chest into the center of the triangle that you made with your hands.

Breathe in one, two, three, four on the way down, and breathe out one, two on the way up.

*Dumbbell Shoulder Press (Shoulders, also assisted by Triceps)

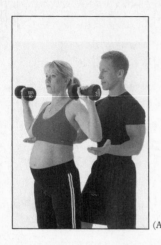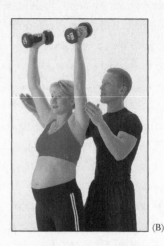

(A)　　　　　　　　(B)

(A) Position: Stand in good posture, holding a dumbbell in each hand up at shoulder level with your palms facing inward.

(B) Movement: Press the dumbbells straight up over your head while rotating your palms outward away from you. Lift them up until the dumbbells almost touch, but do not completely lock your elbows. Then lower the weights back down to the starting position.

Breathe out one, two on the way up, and breathe in one, two, three, four on the way down.

*Lateral Flyes (Shoulders)

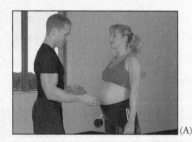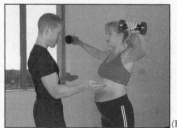

(A)　　　　　　　　(B)

(A) Position: Stand in good posture, holding a dumbbell in each hand down by your legs with your palms facing in toward you.

(B) Movement: Slightly bend your elbows and, using your shoulder muscles, lift your arms out away from your body. Lift up until your hands are at about eye level. Hold the weight there for a count of one, then slowly lower the weight back down to the starting position.

Breathe out one, two on the way up, and breathe in one, two, three, four on the way down.

Caution: Maintain good posture throughout the entire movement, and do not swing or lift the weight using momentum.

*Bent Flyes (Rear Shoulders)

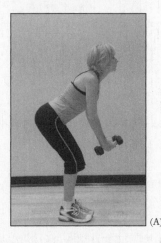 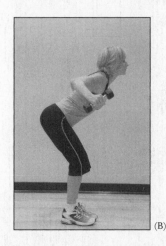

(A) (B)

(A) Position: Hold a dumbbell in each hand down by your legs with your palms facing in toward your body. Bend forward, keeping your head up, your back in lifting posture, and your knees bent until your chest is just above parallel with the floor.

(B) Movement: Raise the dumbbells up and away from your body by pulling up and out with your elbows until the weights are in line with your shoulders. At the top of the movement, squeeze your

shoulder blades together for a count of two before slowly lowering them back down to the starting point.

Breathe out one, two on the way up, and breathe in one, two, three, four on the way down.

Tip: This is a great movement for overcoming computer-posture damage. It builds up the muscles in your lower back.

Caution: Do not bend over too far or straighten your legs out, or you may strain your lower back. Also, as always, do not use momentum by lifting your body up in order to lift the weight.

*Reverse Grip Pulldown (Back)

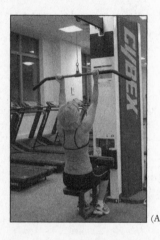
(A)

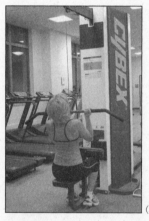
(B)

(A) Position: Sit in a pull-down machine and reach up under the bar and grip it. Your palms should be facing you, and your arms should be shoulder width apart and stretched up as high as they will go so you are being held down by the kneepads.

(B) Movement: Pull the bar all the way down to the sternum, right below your collarbone, and hold for a count of two. Do this while squeezing your shoulder blades and shoulders together with your back muscles before going back to the starting position. During the movement, stay in good posture, with your head up and an arch in your lower back.

Breathe out one, two on the way up, and breathe in one, two, three, four on the way down.

Tip: Reverse grips let you get more range of motion out of your back muscles.

Caution: Do not lean back too far during the movement or use your body to swing the weight down.

*Front-Grip Pulldown (Back)

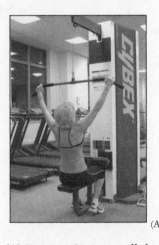 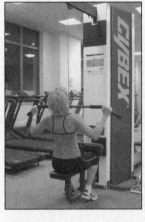

(A)   (B)

(A) Position: Sit in a pull-down machine and reach up over the bar and grip it. Your palms should be facing away from you, and your arms should be three to six inches beyond shoulder width apart and stretched up as high as they will go so you are being held down by the knee pads.

(B) Movement: Pull the bar all the way down to your sternum, right below your collarbone, and hold for a count of two. Do this while squeezing your shoulder blades and shoulders together with your back muscles before going back to the starting position. During the movement, stay in good posture, with your head up and an arch in your lower back.

Breathe out one, two on the way up, and breathe in one, two, three, four on the way down.

Caution: A popular way to do pulldowns is to pull the bar behind your neck. You should avoid this type of pulldown as it creates bad posture and can hurt your neck.

One-Arm Dumbbell Row (Back)

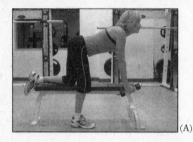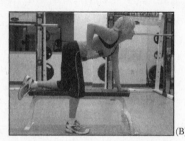

(A)   (B)

(A) Position: Holding a dumbbell in one hand, place the opposite hand and the opposite knee on a bench. Bend over so your torso is parallel with the floor, while keeping your head up and the weightlifter's arch in your lower back.

(B) Movement: Reach out in front of you with the weight and then, using your back lateral muscles, pull your elbow back and up as far as it will go. Hold this lift for a count of one at the top, and then slowly lower it until you are reaching out with the weight again. When you are finished, switch hands and leg positions.

Breathe out one, two on the way up, and breathe in one, two, three, four on the way down.

Tip: Try to focus on your back by really feeling as if you are rowing.

Caution: Do not use momentum to lift the weight, let your head drop, or round your back.

*Pull-Ups/Chin-Ups (Back)

(A) Position: Hang from a bar with your hands three to six inches greater than shoulder width apart and your palms facing away from

you in order to do a pull-up, or with your hands shoulder width apart and your palms facing you in order to do a chin-up.

(B) Movement: Simply pull your chin up over the bar, hold for a count of one, and then lower yourself down all the way.

Breathe out one, two on the way up, and breathe in one, two, three, four on the way down.

Tip: To help yourself get extra reps, you can put your feet up on a chair or bench or have someone help you up by holding your feet. When you begin to fail, use your legs as leverage.

19 | Training Programs

Having a baby to take care of with his or her own demanding schedule may limit when you can actually fit your training in, especially for single moms and those who work full time outside of the home. While there may be better times than others to exercise, you will have to work out a program of weekly resistance and aerobic Exercise by God that best meets your individual schedule.

Once your baby is older, it will be easier to schedule an exact time for your workouts each day. When that happens, you can note that the healthiest time to exercise is two to three hours following a meal. The best time for burning fat and making changes in your body most quickly is in the morning, before you have eaten anything. But for now, the best time to exercise is anytime you can fit it in. It is important to fit training into your day whenever you can versus not at all.

 I discipline my body like an athlete, training it to do what it should.

—1 Corinthians 9:27

Training Schedule

Women should focus on doing two lower-body resistance workouts per week and one upper-body resistance workout. You can safely do fat-burning aerobics anywhere from two to six days a week. If your aerobic session is very intense, you should limit this activity to three or four times per week to avoid injury.

Also, your muscles typically need five to six days to recover, so if you have an extremely intense upper- or lower-body workout, make sure you take the appropriate time between workouts.

Seven-Day Women's Basic Health and Body-Shaping Schedule

One lower-body resistance routine
One upper-body resistance routine
Two to three aerobic activities
Two rest days

Day 1: Lower Body
Day 2: Aerobic
Day 3: Upper Body
Day 4: Rest
Day 5: Aerobic
Day 6: Rest or Aerobic
Day 7: Rest
(Repeat)

Seven-Day Women's Accelerated Health and Body-Shaping Schedule

Two lower-body resistance routines
One upper-body resistance routine
At least three aerobic activities
One to two rest days

Two Rest Days

    Day 1: Lower Body

    Day 2: Aerobic

    Day 3: Upper Body

    Day 4: Rest

    Day 5: Aerobic

    Day 6: Lower Body and Aerobic

    Day 7: Rest

    (Repeat)

One Rest Day

    Day 1: Lower Body

    Day 2: Aerobic

    Day 3: Upper Body

    Day 4: Aerobic

    Day 5: Lower Body

    Day 6: Aerobic

    Day 7: Rest

    (Repeat)

Quick-Set Resistance Programs

The Body by God recommends quick-set programs, which allow you to get in a workout for an individual body part in as little as three minutes. You can easily find three minutes with any baby's schedule, and you can create significant changes by reducing body-fat percentage and increasing muscle tone. The routines that follow are the ultimate way to perform resistance training. They are short and simple, and you can use them to increase the intensity of your workouts, shorten your workout times, and speed up your results safely.

Types of Quick Sets

Decline Set
- Pick one exercise, and do it for eight to twelve repetitions until failure.
- Rest five to six seconds.
- Lower the weight five to twenty pounds and do the exercise again for six to eight repetitions until failure.
- Rest five to six seconds.
- Lower the weight five to twenty pounds again, and do another six to eight repetitions until failure.

Pause Set
- Pick one exercise, and do it for eight to twelve repetitions until failure.
- Rest five to six seconds.
- Using the same weight, do the exercise again until failure.
- Rest five to six seconds.
- Repeat this process until you cannot do the exercise for more than one to two repetitions.

Monster Set
- Pick one exercise and perform it using the Decline Set or the Pause Set.
- Do not rest and begin to perform a *different* exercise for *another* body part using the Decline or Pause Set.

Note: The other body part should be one that is not used while performing the first exercise.

Example: First exercise your chest and biceps, and then exercise your quadriceps and hamstrings.

Monster Sets are combined with a Decline or Pause Set so you can get a tremendously effective workout done in a very short amount of time. For example, after you perform a Pause Set with the Incline Flye Press for your chest, you can immediately begin performing a Decline Set with Hammer Curls for your biceps.

Cycle Set (One Cycle = Three to Six Minutes)
- Set up three to six exercises for the same or different body parts.
- Complete one exercise until failure.
- Immediately begin the next exercise and continue until you have completed all of the three to six exercises you have chosen.
- Continue this pattern (going around the circuit) two to four times.

Example: Choose an exercise for quadriceps, hamstrings, and calves. Do one quadriceps exercise, then one hamstrings exercise, and then one calf exercise. Repeat this circuit two to four times. If you choose more than three exercises, simply add them into the sequence.

Note: You can also set up three exercises for only one body part and go around the circuit if you choose.

Help Reps

Help reps can be used with an Intensity Set. A Help Rep is performed when a helper or spotter stands near you during your set, and when you reach failure that person helps you to perform one or two more repetitions.

Sample Workouts

Decline and Pause Sets allow you to complete an exercise for a particular body part in approximately three minutes. Therefore, a workout consisting of one exercise per body part for three body parts would take only ten minutes, which includes setup time. Workouts become three minutes longer or shorter as you do more or fewer body parts.

One-Day Sample Upper-Body Workout
Three-Minute Body Parts for Six Parts (Twenty-Minute Workout)

Chest and bicep workout together, using the Monster Set format
- Incline Dumbbell Flye Press / Decline Set with Barbell Curl / Pause Set

Triceps and abdominal workout together, using the Monster Set format
- One-Arm Triceps Extension / Decline Set with Abdominal Crunch / Decline Set
- Do crunches using a weight behind the head (or Pause Set if you are unable to use weight)

Back and shoulder workout together, using the Monster Set format
- Front Pulldowns / Decline Set with Lateral Flyes / Decline Set

One-Day Sample Lower-Body Workout
Three-Minute Body Parts for Three Parts (Ten-, Twenty-, and Thirty-Minute Workouts)

For Ten-Minute Workout
Quadriceps and hamstring workout together, using the Monster Set format
- One-Legged Squat / Decline Set with Straight-Leg Dead Lift / Pause Set

Calves
- One-Legged Calf Raise / Decline Set

For Twenty-Minute workout, add:
- Lunge / Decline Set with Leg Extensions / Pause Set
- Seated Calf Raises / Pause Set

For Thirty-Minute workout, add:
- Abduction and Adduction / Decline Set with Hamstring Curls / Decline Set
- Squats / Decline Set with Hamstring Curls / Decline Set
- Standing Calf Raise / Decline Set

Or: Ten- or Fifteen-Minute Lower-Body Cycle Set
- One-Legged Squat *then* Hamstring Curl *then* One-Legged Calf Raise (Go around three or four times for ten or fifteen minutes.)

For Twenty- or Thirty-Minute Cycle Set
- One-Legged Squat *then* Straight-Leg Dead Lift *then* Seated Calf Raise *then* Leg Extension *then* Hamstring Curl *then* One-Legged Calf Raise (Go around three or four times for twenty or thirty minutes.)

 Combining Aerobics and Resistance Training

Perform the following exercises three to five times a week for fifteen minutes with a five-minute warm-up and cool-down phase.
- Walking with ankle or hip weights while doing shoulder, bicep, and triceps movements (combines all three muscle groups)
- Walking with ankle or hip weights while holding hand weights and doing shoulder, bicep, and triceps movements (combines all three)
- Doing an aerobics class that uses hand weights while stepping, lunging, and/or bending at the knees (combines all three)

- Doing yard or housework that requires both leg and arm motions (combines all three as long as there are at least fifteen minutes of straight activity)
- Riding a stationary piece of cardio equipment that has foot and arm pedals (combines all three)
- Swimming (combines all three)

▲ ▲ ▲

20 | Fitting Movement into Your Schedule

God has given mothers a very important role in life, and even though He never allows anyone more than she can handle, moms often feel they have a bit too much! The truth of the matter is that mothers have very challenging and full lives juggling their families, their households, their careers, and themselves. But it is *because* a mother's life is so busy and full that she needs to fit movement into her schedule. This way she can keep fit and healthy for the others she must care for. She also needs exercise simply to have the energy to get through her day's obligations.

Just like shopping, haircuts, doctors' appointments, and housework, exercise needs to be scheduled. If possible, schedule it for first thing in the morning. This way you do it before everything else, and you are less likely to put it off, be too tired, or not have time for it later. Also, by doing it first thing in the morning, you are saying, *My health is a priority.* This sets a great example for all those around you.

Morning is the best time for me. I schedule time for God and time for exercise every morning. I go to great lengths to stick to this and work everything else around it, even if it means I have to get up at 4:00 AM.

If the morning doesn't work for you for some reason, try scheduling exercise during lunchtime, naptime, or after work. If for some reason I can't run in the morning due to a lot of phone appointments, I will hop on my elliptical trainer while I'm on the phone.

Whatever works best is fine. The goal is simply to make the time, no matter when it is. And if all else fails and you don't find that half-hour or hour you need, be sure to work in several mini-workouts. Just be on the lookout for movement opportunities—ten minutes here and there are better than doing nothing. Walk as much as you can: to the park, to the store, to your friends' homes. Leave the car in the garage, and move your body the way God had planned.

It's all a matter of planning and priorities. If movement is a big enough priority, you *will* find the time. One of the best ways to make it a priority is to write down your short- and long-term fitness goals. Having a plan makes goals easier to achieve, and it has been proven that written goals are more likely to be accomplished.

Tips for Scheduling Movement

- Be aware of the time. You typically know when your child eats, sleeps, and plays. Schedule your exercise around those times.

- Choose activities that you can take your child along on, such as jogging with a stroller.

- Use home exercise equipment or aerobic exercise tapes you enjoy while your child is napping.

- Join an aerobics class that allows you to bring your child to the nursery.

- Do shorter workouts. Whenever you have five or ten minutes, put them to good use. Climb the stairs, jump rope, or do some quick sets with your weights.

- Enlist the help of family or friends. Share babysitting times with friends or ask family to help for a block of time each day. A grandmother or aunt might love this time.

- Be flexible! Your days are no longer your own, but when an hour or half-hour is yours, be ready.

Forty-Day Plan for Movement

Your goal should be to incorporate your fitness program into your life each day for forty days. By doing this you should be able to get 40 percent better for God during that time. If you can faithfully do your exercises for these forty days, you will find that you have created a new habit, and it will be easier for you to continue with this new, healthy lifestyle. Make movement an important part of your life, and God will reward you for your commitment by giving you a healthier body in which to live.

God has no physical body—no physical presence in this world—except through His people. If His people take even miniscule steps toward becoming healthier in mind, body, and spirit, God will meet them more than halfway and transform them into the shining examples of His love that He always intended them to be.

Transformation, however, does not occur without pain and sacrifice. Change comes hard for some people because it's easier to keep doing things the way we've always done them. Change means work, and most of us don't like that! Because God made us, He knows that. So if we want to become people God can use to change the world, we need to become more like Him.

Most of us could not handle an immediate, one-time 40 percent change in every area of our lives. But changing 1 percent each day for forty days is easy! Eating Food by God, exercising the Body by God, and sharpening the Soul and Spirit by God by managing your time and stress results in a person God can better use to help others.

Don't lose sight of my words. Let them penetrate deep within your heart, for they bring life and radiant health to anyone who discovers their meaning.
—**Proverbs 4:21–22**

PART V | Stress Management by God for Moms

21 | Peace by God for Moms

As I shared with you in Part III, when I was a teenager I incurred stress daily by going to the gym, being weighed, and then facing indifference from my coaches. Did I recognize it as stress? No, not at the time, but my body *did*. It responded to this stress and expressed itself as an upset stomach, digestive problems, and the inability to eat. My body endured large degrees of stress when I was a young girl, which unfortunately I cannot go back and change.

I can, however, make sure that stress does not get out of hand *today*. Whatever amount of stress you endured previously is now in the past too. As I did, you have the ability to change your present and future.

After recognizing the stress I endured for years and the effects it had on my body, I worked hard to obtain healthier habits so that my Body by God would be strong enough to handle anything. I ate better, exercised, prayed, and read my Bible daily. I learned the art of being very organized and efficient with my time. I pretty much mastered juggling work, running a household, and having relationships with my husband and with God. Yes, there were times when a monkey wrench was thrown into the cogwheel, but I seemed to handle it much better than I had before.

This, however, all changed when Nicole was born. This one tiny human being, who weighed less than ten pounds, immediately changed my entire life. I've mentioned that I no longer seemed to be able to juggle all of the things I had previously. Because Nicole was so demanding of my time, I could no longer complete all the tasks for which I was responsible. This made me feel not only stressed, but incompetent! How could one tiny baby keep me from completing even one-third of all that I had before? Many of my patients were mothers, and none of them seemed to be as stressed as I was—or so I thought. Why couldn't I handle everything? I expected more of myself!

The truth of the matter is that most new mothers experience an initial feeling of stress and incompetence. We must go through a period of adjustment. Unfortunately, just because we finally make it through the transition period doesn't mean that stress stops. Mothers simply have stress; it's a fact of life.

There is stress when babies won't stop crying and go to sleep, when you drop them off at day care for the first time, when you attempt to potty-train them, and when they stumble and fall. There is stress on their first day of school and every day after that while watching them grow, learn, and make mistakes. Some of these days will be filled with good stress, but some will be days of bad stress. (I will define how to tell the difference between good stress and bad a few pages ahead.)

The key is to stop the bad stress and get it under control as soon as you can. You can't eliminate stress from your life altogether, as much as you'd like to, so you must find a way to deal with reducing its negative effects on your Body by God.

The Dangers of Stress on Your Body by God

Many say that stress is *all in our heads*. My response is that they're partially correct. The more accurate statement would be that stress is *in our heads* and *in our bodies!*

Stress is real. It *isn't* something we fabricate in our minds. It's a real response to *outside* stimuli that affects our *insides*—our mental state *and* our physical state. Everyone has stress to some degree. It's a natural response to tension caused by demands and pressures in life. It is only when this tension exceeds your body's comfort level that it affects you in a negative way. When this happens, you need to nip it in the bud before it does damage to your Body by God. Stress is also a major cause of spinal misalignments called subluxation. Regular chiropractic adjustments will correct subluxations before they can cause damage to vital organs.

As a new mother, you now face a whole new set of challenging situations that may cause additional stress in your life. This may push you to a level that exceeds your body's ability to handle stress effectively. It is at this point when it becomes dangerous. Stress affects your nervous system, digestive system, organs, and more. The real problem is that you most likely will not immediately see or feel all the damage that your stress is causing, so you may ignore the source. As a silencer works on a gun, you may not hear the shot fired, but it can still cause you serious pain or kill you.

According to the U.S. Center for Disease Control and Prevention, more than $1 billion per year is spent on health care for stress-related illnesses. Physicians state that 75 percent of their patients seek help for stress-related health issues. The damage that stress causes adds up over time and accumulates within your body. This results in, directly and indirectly, numerous types of illness, disorders, and your inability to fight disease.

Fight-or-Flight Response

When your Body by God faces a threat, your *sympathetic nervous system* (SNS) responds as a fireman responds to an alarm. Your SNS sends out signals to your body that force it to prepare for *fight* or *flight*. Your adrenal glands excrete the hormone adrenaline, which prepares your body to take on the perceived threat.

In the Bible, young David's body certainly went into a fight-or-flight mode when he came face-to-face with Goliath. But today it doesn't take a nine-foot giant to send your body into stress mode. It may take only a traffic jam, a crying baby, or a noise in the middle of the night that awakens you.

In smaller degrees, this response is triggered on a continuous basis by work, daily pressures, and lifestyle. Unfortunately, uncontrolled stress causes the body to be too often in this state, which was designed to protect your body in emergencies. This destructive state is damaging to your Body by God, and this destruction is cumulative—the damage does add up over time.

▶ Caution: Don't Ignore Stress

Stress is not imagined. It is real and causes real damage to your body. It produces emotional distress and has a negative impact on your entire Body by God.

Physical Damage Stress Causes

Following are some of the physical responses to stress:

Organs

When you feel stress, the first response occurs within your brain, which immediately sends out signals to various parts of your body. Your lungs, heart, and digestive system are some of the organs affected.

A change in your breathing rate takes place. It increases, causing additional oxygen to enter your bloodstream. This added oxygen, along with your increased breathing rate, can then cause dizziness and even hyperventilation.

Your blood flow also changes under stress. Overstimulation and an increased blood flow affect some organs, while an understimulation and decrease of blood flow take place in others. The blood flow to your heart increases, making your heart pump harder and faster. This can result in heart palpitations and chest pain. If this response happens over and over again, it can lead to an increased risk for heart attacks, strokes, and artery blockages.

A decreased blood flow occurs within your digestive tract. Blood flow shifts away from your digestive system, causing it to slow down. Your stomach, intestines, spleen, and kidneys can all be affected, resulting in symptoms of indigestion, constipation, or diarrhea. Untreated, long-term stress can also increase acid production in your stomach and cause ulcers.

This country now produces hundreds of products to mask the effects of digestive disorders. One may stop acid reflux, while another puts an end to indigestion. Popping these "magic" pills may help ease your symptoms temporarily, but it is important to address the *cause* of your symptoms if you want *permanent* relief. Stress may be that cause.

Body Chemistry

Stress can also affect your body's chemistry. Under normal circumstances, the Body by God regulates and maintains normal balances of insulin, estrogen, testosterone, adrenaline, and cholesterol. When stress occurs, however, the brain responds negatively by changing your body's chemistry to meet its current situation. As a result, cells and chemicals get out of balance and transform.

As an example: a stressful situation may cause a surge of hormones or adrenaline to be discharged into the body. A state of hyped-up adrenaline or hormones can create a number of problems. At the lower end of the spectrum there is sleeplessness, exhaustion, aggression, irritability, moodiness, or headaches. On the other end of the spectrum, it can increase blood pressure, rupture heart muscles, produce blood clots, and cause arteries to close due to plaque buildup. Continuous stress can also lower your immune system's efficiency, making you more susceptible to disease and illnesses.

Physical Effects

Physical (outward) symptoms are a common effect in times of stress as well. How many of us have had sweaty palms as a result of being stressed? Some women may clench their teeth, blush, or break out in hives. Others' mouths might become dry, making swallowing difficult; muscles may tighten, causing back pain; and the skin may react by triggering an acne or cold-sore breakout. Your responses may be different, but your body *is* responding.

Aging is another physical effect of stress. It may manifest as wrinkles, skin discoloration, changes in hair or nails, and other factors associated with the typical aging process. I have met patients I thought were in their fifties or sixties only to find out later they were in their forties. When I got to know them, I found out they experienced great degrees of stress in their lives, which contributed to their aged and haggard look.

Nutrients

As stress permeates your body, it depletes you of valuable nutrients such as vitamins, minerals, and amino acids. Insufficient supplies of these nutrients are dangerous, because they are essential for proper body function. This depletion has a significant impact on your immune system. A weakened immune system can make you more susceptible to colds, flu symptoms, cold sores, skin problems, and other illnesses. A weakened immune system over an extended period of time due to stress can lead to more serious responses such as cancers and autoimmune and heart diseases.

Your immune system needs to be strongest when your body is in a state of stress. Unfortunately, just the opposite happens, causing your entire Body by God to be placed in a very vulnerable and defenseless state.

Have mercy on me, LORD, for I am in distress. My sight is blurred because of my tears. My body and soul are withering away.

—Psalm 31:9

Types of Stress

Positive Stress (Eustress)

Eustress may be associated with getting married, finding out that you are pregnant, getting your dream job, or winning the lottery. This is a stressful situation that you tend to feel good about and adapt to in a healthy manner.

Negative Stress (Distress)

Distress may be associated with work overload, financial difficulties, a sick child, or a broken relationship. Your body doesn't adapt to negative stress in a healthy manner. Instead it prolongs it and may manifest itself in feelings of failure, anger, or fear.

Physical Stress

Physical stress is a result of exercise or manual labor done too rigorously. Over time, this type of physical activity can be abusive to your joints, muscles, and tendons. You may also experience physical stress by *not* doing any physical activity. Occupations that require long hours of sitting, standing, or assuming unnatural positions can also cause physical stress to your body. Individuals in such situations are prone to negative effects of the chronic wrong use, or lack of use, of their spines, joints, ligaments, and muscles.

Toxic (Chemical) Stress

Smoking, drugs, environmental pollution, toxins in household and personal hygiene products, and chemical-laden foods (as

I discussed in the Food by Man section) can all directly cause something known as *chemical stress*. These toxic elements stress your body and have a negative impact on the health of your Body by God.

Relax. You're in God's Hands

But in my distress I cried out to the LORD; yes, I prayed to my God for help. He heard me from his sanctuary; my cry reached his ears.

—Psalm 18:6

God knew you would have to deal with stress in your life. He knew there would be repercussions to your Body by God if you allowed it to get out of hand. But He also gave you the ability to keep your stress in hand. He gave you the gift of prayer. Romans 8:26 states, "The Holy Spirit helps us in our distress. For we don't even know what we should pray for, nor how we should pray. But the Holy Spirit prays for us with groanings that cannot be expressed in words." When you are so stressed that even burned toast upsets you, you should stop everything you are doing and pray. The Holy Spirit will help you by expressing what you cannot, due to your inability to see the situation clearly.

"LORD, help!" they cried in their trouble, and he rescued them from their distress.

—Psalm 107:6

But most importantly, God gave you the gift of peace. It is through Him that you will find the peace you need in order to deal with your stressful situations, as Mary of Nazareth did in hers.

Mary's Story

Mary's heart was pounding out of her chest. Her breathing had become so shallow that she was almost hyperventilating. Her palms were sweaty, and her stomach felt queasy. She pressed her ear harder up against the door in order to hear Joseph's voice. She knew he was asking her parents for her hand in marriage. As she strained to listen, she heard footsteps coming toward the door and jumped back, almost falling down, to appear as casual as possible.

Her father opened the door and extended his hand. Mary moved closer, put her sweaty hand in his, and was led into the next room where Joseph was waiting. The arrangements had been made. Mary was engaged to Joseph.

What exhilaration Mary felt, and what stress! She was going to marry Joseph! He was such a handsome and good man. Could she be a good wife to him? Could she make him happy? Then her thoughts went to what a wonderful family they would have together. Oh, the wedding! Her thoughts quickly changed. There were preparations to make, her wedding clothes, the cake. There was so much to do.

Mary's mind was supercharged as adrenaline pumped through her veins. She was in a state of eustress. Even though it was obvious that her body was physically reacting to this stress, it was created by a wonderful event and positive situation, which allowed her body to adapt to it in a healthy manner.

It wasn't much later when Mary was startled by a visitor at her door.

"Gabriel appeared to her and said, 'Greetings, favored woman! The Lord is with you!'

Confused and disturbed, Mary tried to think what the angel could mean. 'Don't be frightened, Mary,' the angel told her, 'for God has decided to bless you! You will become pregnant and have a son, and you are to name him Jesus. He will be very great and will be called the Son of the Most High. And the Lord God will give him the throne of his ancestor David. And he will reign over Israel forever; his Kingdom will never end!'

Mary asked the angel, 'But how can I have a baby? I am a virgin.'

The angel replied, 'The Holy Spirit will come upon you, and the power of the Most High will overshadow you. So the baby born to you will be holy, and he will be called the Son of God'" (Luke 1:28–35).

Mary's mind began to race. She was also a fourteen-year-old girl who was engaged to Joseph. How could she tell him? Joseph would certainly believe that she had been unfaithful to him, and then he couldn't possibly marry her. If others found out she was pregnant, she would be an outcast and disgrace to her family, or worse, stoned to death.

Mary was stressed, but this time it was distress. Her body was not handling the situation well. She felt sick to her stomach and knew that if her stress continued, it would place her body, and the body of the child she was carrying, in a position that was damaging, dangerous, and susceptible to illness and disease.

Yet Mary knew that God knew what was best for her and responded to the angel, "I am the Lord's servant, and I am willing to accept whatever he wants" (Luke 1:38). With these words a new sense of peace washed over her body. Her damaging stress subsided, leaving her calm and prepared for what was ahead.

▲ ▲ ▲

God promised you peace, and if you ask for it, you will receive it. Second Thessalonians 3:16 states, "May the Lord of peace himself always give you his peace no matter what happens. The Lord be with you all." But some of the most comforting words I have found are in John 14:27: "I am leaving you with a gift—peace of mind and heart. And the peace I give isn't like the peace the world gives. So don't be troubled or afraid."

Being a mother gives you numerous opportunities to experience negative stress.

It may come after you haven't slept well for days due to nighttime feedings, and then your baby develops colic and doesn't stop crying. It may come after your child has been ill, and the doctors can't figure out what is wrong. It may come after a hard day at a demanding job, arriving at home to find that you have to make dinner, help with homework, clean the house, do the laundry, and still spend some quality time with your spouse!

Life as a mother is a full-time, demanding job that often comes with stressful times. Thankfully, God wants to give us peace to get through it. His peace helps us cope better, allowing us to deal with all of the situations that we deem stressful. His peace is there for the taking, to help us handle our stress today and tomorrow.

22 | This Is Your Brain with Kids

The way you see the world today is a result of your preprogramming. Every event and situation you have encountered has been gathered, sorted, and then programmed into your mind, just as you would program a computer. From this database that your mind has created will come the interpretation of every event you experience in the future.

Each time you face a new situation, your mind will utilize your database of existing information to help you determine how you *see* and respond to the situation. It will create your perception—your *point of view*. At that time, along with determining your response, you will ascertain whether the situation is positive or negative.

> *Our lives are a fragrance presented by Christ to God. But this fragrance is perceived differently by those being saved and by those perishing.*
> —2 Corinthians 2:15

An analogy of perception is this: Imagine you were wearing glasses with colored lenses. You might wear yellow lenses and see the world one way, and your spouse may wear blue lenses, which makes him see it differently. Perhaps you are planning a family vacation. You would like to go to the beach because you believe it would be a positive and enjoyable experience. You remember your childhood days of making sand castles and wading in the water with your siblings. Your perception from your yellow lenses is *positive* and that the beach would make a wonderful vacation for your young family.

On the other hand, looking through his blue lenses, your husband cringes at the idea. He remembers going to the beach and being sucked under by a wave, almost drowning. Then, not daring to go back into the water, he remembers sitting on the beach while others played and ending up being sunburned to a crisp. His perception of such a vacation is *negative* and that the beach would be a nightmare for your family.

Past experiences created both perceptions. Both persons believe they are correct in their assumptions of how this particular vacation would turn out.

I believe that children are initially born wearing *rose-colored glasses*. If you watch them play, everything is such a joy to them. Watch two children making mud pies. They are having *so* much fun—until their mothers step in. One scolds her child, scoops him up, and rushes him inside to the bathtub. The other mother bends down and begins making mud pies with her child, laughing and having fun.

Do you think each child will continue with the same beliefs about playing in the mud? Initially they shared joy; their perceptions were the same. Due to the different reactions they received from their mothers, however, their perceptions will change, and their future responses will reflect that. One child has just switched from rose-colored glasses in this situation to brown-colored ones due to the new information that was just programmed into his database.

Many people would love to be able to see the world through a child's eyes—ones that have not been programmed with negativity. The good news is that you *can* switch glasses, and like a computer, you can upgrade and reprogram. You *can* change your perception.

Why is this so important in a segment on stress? Because situations don't become stressful until your perception of them deems that they should be. You determine, every minute of the day, whether or not each event that takes place is positive or negative and causes you stress or not.

Creation of Perception

Various factors, such as your history, culture, goals, and self-esteem, can influence your perception of situations. Let's explore these areas further.

History

Past experiences with people, events, education, conflicts, and other situations will determine almost 90 percent of your current beliefs and perceptions toward present events.

- When Noah tried to warn the people of the great flood that was coming, no one believed him. This was partly due to their historic beliefs and experiences. They had never seen a flood because until then it had never rained. They didn't believe that one was possible; therefore, their perception was that it would not happen.

- If you had a stay-at-home mom growing up and chose to be the same for your child, you may not understand how your best friend could go back to a forty-hour work week when her baby was just six weeks old. You are not programmed to understand this. On the other hand, she may have grown up loving day care, with so many other children to play with, and might not understand keeping your baby home with no playmates. Each woman's programming is different due to past experiences.

- Your perception might be that your child would get the best education and have the most enjoyable experience in a private school. Your best friend might believe that private school isn't necessary and public school would give her child a better, more positive experience. Both of you believe something different, and most likely it was due to your past experience with your own schooling and teachers or those of people you knew.

Culture

Your mother, father, siblings, grandparents, and other relatives pass down your culture to you. Your occupation, friends, geographic area, school, and religion influence it. Different cultures play an important role in how you behave, believe, work, and treat people.

- If you grew up in China, your perception might be that having a male child is better than having a female, and that having more than two children is bad because it is punishable by extra taxes.
- If you grew up in a family that hugged and kissed everyone all the time, your perception would be that this is normal and positive. If, however, you grew up in a family that didn't express love in this manner, you might find such expressions uncomfortable and a negative experience for you.
- Religions can create major differences in cultural perceptions. All you have to do is look at the differences in beliefs between a Christian and a Muslim. This also applies to geographic areas. Growing up in America, I believe we have a good country and feel positive about it. If, however, I grew up in Iraq, I might believe that this country is evil and see it in a negative light.

Culture greatly influences perceptions because we rely not only on our own personal histories to create data for the mind's database, but we also include the data of generations before ours. We include data from those who live around us, attend the same churches, and have the same education. We rely on their histories and information and add them to our databases.

Goals

The intensity of your desires will have an effect on your perceptions.

- You may be a very meticulous person, keeping everything neat, tidy, and in order. Your perception is that this is the most efficient way to achieve your goals, and it bothers you when others do not conduct their lives in this manner. As a result, you might find your husband's sloppiness and disorder very upsetting. He, on the other hand, might not see anything wrong with it because the two of you have been programmed differently.

- You may have a desire to save the money you earn and accumulate wealth in order to take care of your family. You will do the things necessary to accomplish this and see them as positive steps to achieving your goals. Your neighbor might believe that you should live for the day and spend what you have because you may not be here tomorrow. He will live his life in a manner that reflects his goals. You might see his actions as negative and yours as positive, while he might see them in reverse.

Everyone has different goals in life, but it is your desire to achieve them that will dictate your actions. Your perception regarding those actions will be created in a manner that is complementary to what you need in order to achieve your goals.

Self-Esteem

How you see yourself will influence your future. It will determine how you interact with others, what you *believe* you are capable of doing, what you will *attempt* or not attempt to do in life, and in what manner or at what level you will do it.

- If your self-esteem is low and you believe you are not worthy to be loved, you might choose poor relationships with people who do not love you. If, however, you believe you deserve a strong, lifelong love, you will most likely choose to be with an individual who will fill those shoes.

Changing Your Programming

All of your thoughts, words, and actions are limited and created by the database of knowledge that causes your perceptions. You could call it your *perception programming*. Changing, upgrading, or deleting this programming, however, is often necessary. It is important that you don't become so attached to your perceptions that they are inflexible, causing you to judge people and situations before knowing all the real facts.

- For example, all the women in your family and extended family have had children. To you this is expected of married women. Now your sister tells you that she doesn't want to have children, and instead wants to pursue her career and travel the world. Your perception programming can't even begin to comprehend how she could think like this. You might feel as though she is selfish and passing on her life's purpose. You pass judgment on her before she has even had a chance to explain or show you what she can accomplish in other areas of her life.
- In another example, you might see a young pregnant girl. Your perception programming might respond negatively; you think the girl has been promiscuous and irresponsible. You might find her repulsive and judge her in a negative way. But what if this girl happened to be a fifteen-year-old who was raped at knifepoint, who didn't believe in abortion and took on the burden of carrying the child to give it up

for adoption? You didn't have all of the facts. You perceived the situation one way and judged it accordingly.

The Bible is very clear on judging others. Matthew 7:2 states, "For others will treat you as you treat them. Whatever measure you use in judging others, it will be used to measure how you are judged." God is the only one who knows all that affects each of our lives. Since you can never stand in a person's shoes long enough to know, *your* perceptions can't be used to pass judgment on another.

Stop judging others, and you will not be judged.
—Matthew 7:1

But just as we might judge other people, we also judge situations. In every situation we face, our perception programming clicks on, sorts through the data we have inputted, and calculates a response. It is up to you to recognize whether the data is good or might be limited and need upgrading. If you find that old perceptions no longer apply, that data should be eliminated entirely.

Your preprogramming might tell you that the following situations should cause you negative stress: attending a public event, speaking to your boss, being around a dog, or riding an elevator, to name a few. Everyone has situations programmed in her mind as being stressful. Reprogramming takes looking at each situation in a new light (or with different lenses). You must analyze your thoughts, emotions, and reactions and determine if they best suit the situation and your needs. If not, you can begin to reprogram your perceptions and replace them with positive, nonstressful responses.

A Self-Inflicted Wound

Stress and motherhood seem to go hand in hand, but it doesn't have to be that way. While some degree of stress is not entirely avoidable, it is controllable. Many women feel they are victimized by stress on a daily basis, but if that's the case, it's because they are allowing this to happen.

When you face potentially stressful situations, you have control. You have the ability to choose to react to the situation with stress, thereby inflicting the results of stress on your body; or you have the ability to control your thoughts and not respond in a stressful manner.

▶ Note: Stress Is Different for Everyone
Not everyone perceives and interprets the same situations as stressful. The individual's reaction to the situation—not the situation itself—determines his or her response.

Imagine a morning like this: After feeding the baby, Mom prepares breakfast for her toddler (Junior). Her husband has to leave the house early for an important meeting at the office and cannot watch the children the way he typically does while Mom showers and dresses. So after Dad leaves, Mom makes sure the baby is in her bed napping and Junior is playing safely while watching *Sesame Street*. She showers and dresses and returns to the kitchen to find Junior playing with the dog. Unfortunately, in Dad's haste to get to the office in time, he forgot to walk the dog, and the dog has had an accident on the kitchen floor. Junior is sitting in it.

This mother has two choices: She can react negatively, causing her stress, *or not*. She can choose to feel victimized and very angry with her husband for not walking the dog, irritated at the dog for the accident, and upset with her child for sitting in it. This would be a situation full of negative stress.

Or this mother can choose not to allow herself to become stressed by the situation and take control over her reaction. Junior was going to have his bath anyway, the dog already did what he had to do so can wait a bit before going out again, and the floor already needed washing! It's all in a day's work!

In this case, if Mom became stressed, she would find it easy and justifiable to blame Dad, the dog, or Junior for her stress. But the truth of the matter is that *no* person on this earth can *make* you feel stressed. *Only you have the power to do that.*

Is Your Cup Half Full or Half Empty?

There are the *haves* and the *have-nots* in life. I'm sure you could place most people you know in one category or the other. The *haves* are those who have so much positive energy and happiness that they seem to bubble over and touch the lives of others in a life-giving way. The *have-nots* appear always to be drained from negativity, stress, and unhappiness. Because they have nothing left to give to others, they instead feed upon the positive energy from those around them. Like a vortex, they suck in all the positive energy they can; yet it is never enough, and they cannot get their fill.

What's the difference between these two groups of people? The *haves* choose to control their responses and react in a nonstressful manner, allowing them to perceive life as positive—their cups are *half full*. The *have-nots* allow stress to take control, creating negative responses—seeing their cups as *half empty*.

Even if you look at only a portion of what God has given you, you will find that your life is not just half full—it is overflowing with blessings.

You prepare a feast for me in the presence of my enemies. You welcome me as a guest, anointing my head with oil. My cup overflows with blessings.

—Psalm 23:5

When you stop focusing on the one small area of distress in your life and take time to look at the big picture, you will find things aren't as bad as you had originally thought. You can focus on the damaged bumper of your car after a fender bender, or you can focus on the fact that no one was harmed. The bumper will cause you negative stress, but realizing that no one was hurt will cause you peace and relief. Which would you choose?

When you start to become more aware and critical of your responses, you will give yourself an opportunity to choose peace and positive thoughts over stress and negative thoughts.

Focus on Others *and* Me?

You now know the importance of focusing on having a cup half full, not half empty, to help alleviate stress. But you might not realize the importance of focusing on yourself as much as you do others. New mothers often fall into the trap of expending so much time on their new babies and everyone else that they quickly dismiss any thoughts of focusing on themselves. Go back to the analogy of the airplane and oxygen mask: you must first put your mask on so that you can help others. If you give and give and never take any time for yourself, you will place your body in a situation where stress can begin to build and take its toll.

Taking time for yourself is not as selfish as you might think. It actually helps you deal with stress better. When you take care of yourself, you are more relaxed and therefore respond more calmly and positively. When your responses are calmer and more positive, you deal more kindly with others, especially your children. When your children receive positive responses from you, they in turn will handle situations more positively. It is a chain that flows from one person to the next. When negativity enters the chain, the chain changes and becomes negative and must be broken. You need to be aware of any negative response that enters your chain of responses and eliminate it; replace it with a positive response.

Mushed Vegetables and Your Brain

Dealing with all the information in this book may seem overwhelming to you right now. Don't worry; it will get easier. A new mother often feels as if her brain has turned to mush. Your language has probably converted to baby talk by now. Your important meetings of the day are with your pediatrician, with whom you will discuss bowel movements, and your schedule is now focused on feedings and naptime. If your brain doesn't feel like mush, it's a miracle!

The telltale sign that your brain has made its final transition over to *mushland* is when you go out to dinner with friends and you don't know what's happening in the world. You realize the only thing you have thought about for the past six weeks is your baby. The real scary moment, however, is when you realize it hasn't only been the past six weeks, but the past six years!

Your brain may never be the same once you have children, but this doesn't have to be negative. You now have an opportunity to open up your mind to many more moments of learning. You now have the opportunity to see situations through a child's eyes—innocent eyes with no preprogrammed perceptions. This will help you to better analyze your current responses and change any negative ones. This is a chance to expand your thinking and change your perceptions. Discard those that are no longer useful and upgrade those that need to be converted from negative to positive, and get help to do so if you need it.

23 | Mother's Guidelines for Peace Management

As we have seen in the previous chapter, stress comes from *your reactions,* not the *actions* of others or from circumstances. No one can make you stressed out except you. It follows then that your own lack of management skills to handle the stresses in your life is the heart of the problem. You alone have the power to change your perceptions, your attitudes, your spin on things. The best way to reduce stress is to take control of your peace, but you cannot do that until you actually have it. So how do you get peace in the first place, so you can control it?

Actually, your peace is sitting on a shelf in heaven, wrapped and tied up with a red ribbon, with your name on the gift tag. It's a big box and there's an abundant supply inside, enough to last your life-time. It was purchased and paid for by God Himself, at a tremendous price, and He's waiting for you to accept it. That's all you have to do: just reach out to God and receive His peace. (Joy, love, grace, and a few other things are there all wrapped and waiting for you, too, also bought and paid for by God.)

When Nicole was three months old, my girlfriend and I planned an Alaskan cruise for our families to take together. She had a five-month-old baby and a fifteen-month-old toddler. At the time I thought this was a wonderful idea, but I had no concept of what I was in for. As the date of our trip got closer, the stress began mounting.

First, I had no idea what to pack for us. Clothing was one thing, but then I worried about somewhere for Nicole to sleep. Should I bring a portable bed? Would I need a car seat and a stroller? Then there was the issue of milk. My mother was going to join us on the trip so that Ben and I could take his son, Skylar, on a few hikes during the stops the cruise makes. Because I was breast-feeding, I wanted to make sure that I would have enough milk for Nicole while I was gone, so I began pumping and freezing milk for her.

The day of the trip arrived and there our two families stood, with seventeen pieces of luggage, waiting for the van to pick us up and take us to the airport. It didn't arrive. After fifteen minutes my husband called the service only to find that they had scheduled our pickup on the wrong day. This added to my stress and made us almost miss our flight. Then I faced a nine-hour flight and a four-hour train ride before even reaching the ship for the cruise!

Of course, no one on the plane wanted to sit next to our families with three small children, and who could blame them? It was stressful enough for me—why spread it to everyone around us?

By the time we finally reached our destination, I was stressed beyond measure. As I unpacked I realized that all of the breast milk that I had pumped and frozen had thawed out. I thought it was ruined, and in the accumulation of my stress I sat on the bed and cried my heart out. That was the final straw. I couldn't handle any more.

At that time, however, Ben came into the room and asked me what was wrong. I told him and his response was, "Worst-case scenario is that we stay on the boat and hang out with the baby so you can breast-feed." He was right. That trip I made the mistake of choosing stress instead of peace. God knew our needs and would take care of us.

The LORD gives his people strength. The LORD blesses them with peace.

—Psalm 29:11

Five Ingredients of Peace by God

I'm going to assume that you've taken my advice and claimed your gift of Peace by God. You've unwrapped your present and now are trying to read the manual that came with it (commonly called *the Bible*). This way you'll know how to make the peace last and to learn how to use it in your daily life. You want to know what peace really is and how it works.

There are five basic ingredients of Peace by God. Once you understand them, you can fully appreciate the tremendous gift God has given you. Let's examine these gifts within the gift that work together to produce peace.

Ingredient #1: Acceptance

If you know that all is well between you and God, your spirit can be at peace. If your spirit (the spiritual part of you) is at peace, your soul (the mind, emotions, and will), and your body (your physical presence in the world) will also be at peace. It's hard for one part to be peaceful by itself because all the parts are inseparable and intertwined.

Peace with God comes from approaching Him on His terms, meeting and knowing Him on a personal basis, recognizing Him as your God, and trusting Him on a moment-by-moment basis for everything you need.

That's a rather simplistic description of a very deep truth, but it will work for our purposes in this book. If you have placed your trust in God, He has accepted you. You are His child, and He loves you and has promised to take care of you. He knows the worst about you, and He loves you anyway. And He has promised that nothing you can do will change that—not ever.

As a mother, you can understand that kind of love. No matter what your child might do, no matter how old he or she is, no matter what you'd like to see changed about him or her, you will always have a mother's love for your child. Multiply that by about a zillion times, and you'll begin to have an inkling of how much God loves you. That's acceptance. You never have to worry about it again. That knowledge generates peace.

To the praise of the glory of his grace, wherein he hath made us accepted in the beloved.

—**Ephesians 1:6** KJV

Ingredient #2: Faith

The letters in the word *faith* stand for the true definition of the word: *Forsaking All, I Trust Him.* Sometimes all you can do is just that: *hang on and trust God.* He does know the end from the beginning, after all, and even the faith to believe in God is a gift from Him. Faith is the engine that drives the train. The train has one car, *fact*, and one caboose, *feeling*. (Notice that feelings are last and least important.) Faith is not based on feelings, it's based on the fact that God has made certain promises to His children and He is not only able to deliver on those promises, He *wants* to do so.

As a mother, you know a lot about faith. You went into labor trusting that the baby would indeed be born. You brought the baby home trusting that you would be able to care for him or her. You feed your baby trusting that the nourishment will cause him or her to grow. Trusting God to help you cope with whatever He allows to come your way each day is an exercise in faith. None of us knows the future for a certainty. But you *can* know the God who holds the future (both yours and your baby's) in His hands. Exercising your faith generates peace.

What is faith? It is the confident assurance that something we want is going to happen. It is the certainty that what we hope for is waiting for us, even though we cannot see it up ahead.

Hebrews 11:1 TLB

Ingredient #3: Love

A mother's love is in a class by itself. Nothing touched the depths of my heart as the love I felt for my daughter as soon as I held her in my arms. The love of God is in a class by itself as well. His love is deeper, stronger, broader, and even more enduring than a mother's love for her baby. The way God loves us is on a totally different plane from human love. His love is eternal, but it is also a *tough* love, pointing out things in our lives we need to attend to for our own good and protecting us from injury and harmful situations by taking us down paths that we don't understand. It is impossible to explain in words both a mother's love and God's love for us. It's enough to know that you are loved: deeply, enduringly, and with great joy on His part. That's a hard concept to grasp, I know, but it's even harder to reject. (Why would anyone want to?)

God's love shows up in our lives through the love we receive from our spouses, our children, our family members, and our friends. Even perfect strangers act lovingly toward us when we get into accidents or something bad happens to us. That, too, is God's love for us in action. Knowing we are loved so well by God contributes to our peace.

There are three things that remain—faith, hope, and love—and the greatest of these is love. Let love be your greatest aim.

—**1 Corinthians 13:13–14:1** TLB

Ingredient #4: Hope

Hope is the thing that keeps you from giving up when all the odds are stacked against you. It's very much like faith, but there are slight differences. Faith carries with it the idea of assurance; hope is more of an expectation or anticipation. Faith confirms that we were *right* in hoping.

What would life be without hope? Terribly discouraging, I

think. Knowing us thoroughly, God created us with the need for something to anticipate. As a mom, you look forward to the events in your baby's life: that first real smile (not a gas bubble!); the first word (it had *better* be Mama or Dada); the first step on those chubby legs; the first day of school; the first two-wheeler; the first home run; the first driver's license; the first date . . . what a wonderful life you are anticipating for your baby!

God doesn't hope, because He *knows*. He doesn't need anticipation, but He knows that *we* do, so He has provided it for us. He has given us every coping tool we need for life's twists and turns, both good and not-so-good. That should give you both hope and peace.

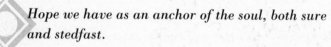

Hope we have as an anchor of the soul, both sure and stedfast.

—Hebrews 6:19 KJV

Ingredient #5: Security

Safety is important to everyone of every age, but as a mother, your primary concern will always be the safety of your child. That concern begins the moment you know you are pregnant and never ends. Safety is just one part of the entire security picture; some of the others are clothing, shelter, food (Food by God, of course!), income, and relationships—all the things we need to feel serene in this world.

But when we leave this world someday (and we all will!), what do we need to feel secure? We won't be able to take our food, shelter, and clothing with us, but we *can* take our relationship with God. And that's really all the security we need, both in heaven and here on earth.

We can know we are secure because God has promised that He will never leave us or forsake us (Heb. 13:5). Security means we don't have a thing to worry about if we have given God control of our lives. Security is having our needs met time after time after time.

Security is knowing that the God who spoke and created the universe loves us and wants us to be happy. Security is knowing that we are abundantly blessed, giving us enough to share with others. Security is great! And it is a huge contributor to peace.

 Because the Lord is my Shepherd, I have everything I need!

—Psalm 23:1 TLB

Take Back Your Peace

There's a popular story about two artists who were asked to paint their conceptions of peace. One painted a tranquil lake at sunrise with mist hovering over the placid water. The other painted a raging torrent of a stream plunging over a waterfall with the storm clouds blackening the sky and the rain pelting down. On the branch of a tree hanging way out over the treacherous water was a bird's nest. In it sat a small bird, hunkered down against the wind and rain, with her eyes shut . . . sleeping. That painting truly illustrated peace: calmness and trust in the middle of the storms of life.

When you focus on stress and give it power over you through your improper reactions, you are not in control. Stress is. That is the opposite of what God intended. You are looking through the wrong end of the telescope. God gave you the power to be peaceful; you have surrendered it by turning around and giving it to others or situations. There's only one thing to do: take it back.

Here's how:

Understand it. Peace is yours for the taking. It means trusting that God is in control, even when it seems that He isn't. Every time you lose your peace, reclaim it. It's always right there waiting.

Accept it. Claim it as yours and practice it every time you feel stressed. It will get easier the more you do it.

Teach it to others. Pass on what you've learned to others who seem stressed. Suggest that they close their eyes for one minute and focus on something that always makes them feel peaceful: a sunset, a beautiful beach, a lazy nap in a hammock under a shade tree. These one-minute vacations really do work!

When life is just too much, when the children are driving you crazy even though you love them to pieces, when you're hit with a diagnosis that scares you, or when you simply just want to crawl into a hole and pull a cover over it . . . your gift of Peace by God is right there within you, waiting for you to use it. It's helpful to think of it as a multimillion dollar savings account that God opened in your name, just sitting there, waiting for you to make withdrawals as you need them. You take what you need at the moment, but there's plenty more where that came from.

PART VI | Time Management by God for Moms

24 | Time by God

And *you* thought the labor was over when you delivered the baby! As you've probably learned by now, the *labor* is just beginning. Motherhood is the art of finding time to do all the things your baby needs you to do, finding time for your husband and/or other children, finding time for yourself, and (if you work outside the home or have a career), finding the strength to go back to work. Oh yes, and finding a way to get your figure back. Sound impossible? If it weren't for God's help, it *would* be.

If anything describes motherhood perfectly, it's this scenario: Years ago there was a man who appeared on various television variety shows with a group of bamboo poles and a stack of dinner plates. He set the poles up in a base so they stood straight up in the air. Then he jiggled them to start them moving. As soon as each one was at the proper speed, he started a dinner plate spinning on top of each pole, moving down the line with lightning speed. By the time he got to the last pole (usually eight to ten poles later), the plate on top of the first pole was just about ready to fall off and crash to the ground. Audiences loved this act! The man looked very calm, but underneath the façade he was frantic. Sound like anyone you know?

Time by Man or Time by God?

God doesn't play favorites: He gave us all the exact same amount of time each day. It's how we manage time that separates the *frantic* from the *fulfilled*. Each of us has 31,536,000 seconds per year. (We get 86,400 more in leap years.) Sounds like a lot when you put it that way! That's the good news. The bad news is that not one of those seconds is retrievable once it's been spent. We have to learn to make each second count because with time, there's no instant replay.

I was in an elevator once in New York City, riding to the top of a forty-eight-story building along with several other people. Two men were talking about their morning routines. One man said, "I only had five minutes, so there wasn't time to do anything. What can you do in just five minutes?" The other man nodded and shrugged his shoulders.

Because in those days New Yorkers didn't talk to strangers in elevators, much less look at them directly, I said nothing. But I was thinking, *What could I do in five minutes? I could save someone's life with CPR; I could walk up a few flights of stairs and get some exercise; I could put a load of clothes in the washer; I could cross off about six little things on my to-do list.* There was no end to what I could have accomplished in five minutes!

More time is not what mothers need; we need to learn to manage what time we have. We can learn to do more in the time we have by being more efficient and determining what's really important. If we cannot manage our time, how can we manage our lives? I learned a lesson that day in the New York elevator: I have all the time I need to do what God has asked me to do. And there's the key to managing your time as a mother.

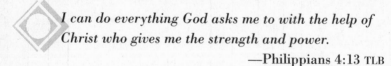

I can do everything God asks me to with the help of Christ who gives me the strength and power.
—Philippians 4:13 TLB

When you became a mother, God made motherhood a priority in your life. That's what He has asked you to do, so He has given you enough time to do whatever it takes to be a good mom. If you're married, He's also given you enough time to invest in your relationship. And He's allotted enough time for you to take care of yourself. (As I pointed out earlier, if you do not take care of yourself, you will eventually not be able to take care of anyone else.)

If you are not managing your time, it's managing you. You are reacting to what life throws at you instead of taking charge of your schedule. Don't feel guilty. It happens to all of us some of the time. The problem comes when it happens every day, month after month. This is management by crisis, not management by God. Management by God is different.

What are the things that are most important to you? Take a piece of paper and answer these questions:

1. What is the thing I would die for if a terrorist made me choose life or it? (We're talking about your values here—faith, freedom, or family, for example.)

2. What do you see as your mission in life (or purpose or call from God)?

3. What is the thing you would like people to remember you for after you die?

The answers to these three questions state your priorities in life—the things you feel are central to who you are and what you'd like to be.

Now here's the fourth and pivotal question:

4. How much of your time is spent on furthering these three areas of your life?

That's the tough one, because it points out where your time is not being spent on the things that matter to you the most.

Time by Man

The Tyranny of the Urgent

The urgencies of life are the things that pop up unexpectedly and demand our attention. Many of the urgencies are good things and deserve attention. But they often keep us focused on what's *good* as opposed to what's *best*. They rob us of our time and, if we allow them to, the urgencies will prevent us from investing our time in the areas of life that are most important to us. Time by God is managing our time to promote health, peace, success, better relationships, and anything else that is good for our futures. We need to choose our priorities according to our most important values. If you begin following some of the guidelines in this book, you will have the time to get your life under control. Don't let *life* manage *you*. It's been said before and bears repeating, that at the end of life, no one says, "I wish I'd spent more time at the office."

 For a man is a slave to whatever controls him.
> —2 Peter 2:19 TLB

Time Zones

ZONE 1 - TIME BY MAN

- Emergency Centered
- Survival Driven
- Reactive Focused

Distractions: *Technology, Hobbies, News & World Events, Treatment for Illness, Emotional Challenges, Fringe Business*

ZONE 2 - TIME BY GOD

- Mission Centered
- Principle Driven
- Cause-Active Focused

▼

> **Missionary Work:** *Healthy Lifestyle, Spiritual Growth, Relationship Building, Social & Community Involvement, Skill Sharpening & New Skill Development, Opportunity, Planning & Organizing, Coaching, Maintenance, Perception Programming*

Time is divided into two zones. Zone 1 represents Time by Man. Zone 2 represents Time by God. To find time for everything in your life, you must discover Time by God.

Zone 1 is focused on survival. Zone 1 energy is spent on our physical, material, intellectual, and emotional needs and desires. Zone 1 behavior is focused on meeting those needs.

Of course we must work to provide our family's and our own basic needs for food, clothing, and shelter. And we usually want to take care of these things in the quickest and easiest ways possible, with as little effort on our part as we can manage—often at the expense of morality, principles, and any thought of how we are affecting those in our spheres of influence. Zone 1 values are material and temporary.

The interesting thing is that the more time you spend on Zone 1 activities, the less time there is for Zone 2. Zone 1 increases and takes over our lives, while Zone 2 shrinks and has less priority. From God's standpoint, this is backward.

So don't worry at all about having enough food and clothing . . . Your heavenly Father already knows perfectly well that you need them, and he will give them to you if you give him first place in your life and live as he wants you to.

—**Matthew 6:31–33** TLB

Zone 2 living is focused on discovering and following your mission in life: how you develop and use the talents God has given you to serve Him and help others. Your mission is why you were given life, why you are here.

Zone 2 behavior is principle driven, with a commitment to morals and ethics. What you do during the day is determined by your commitment to improve your life, reach out to others, and manage your time and your life to bring about success and honor to God. Zone 2 values are spiritual and eternal.

In Zone 2, there are fewer emergencies, and you are focused on the important values in your life (the answers to those three questions I asked you).

In the television series from the sixties and seventies called *The Twilight Zone,* something was always a little *off.* Living in Zone 1 is a bit like that. Whatever amount of effort you expend, no matter how much Zone 1 time you spend in meeting material and immediate needs, your life will always be a bit *off.* In contrast, spending time in Zone 2 in pursuit of a better life puts you in sync with the plan God designed especially for you, which in turn eliminates a lot of stress and wasted time. Investing more time in Zone 2 makes sense, doesn't it?

Taxes, money, cars, houses, interest rates, stocks, politics, clothes, lawsuits, position, scores, place, popularity, appearance, and fear are all part of Time by Man, Zone 1. Charity, love, hope, fairness, honesty, joy, and faith are all characteristics of Time by God, Zone 2. Time spent in Zone 1 focused on the needs of this life may or may not bring you short-term success, but it will produce frustration long term. Time spent in Zone 2 focused on God's needs in preparing yourself and others for eternal life may or may not bring you short-term success as the world thinks of it, but it is guaranteed to bring success and peace long term. You get to choose.

*Don't store up treasures here on earth where they
can erode away or may be stolen. Store them in
heaven where they will never lose their value, and
are safe from thieves. If your profits are in heaven
your heart will be there too.*

—Matthew 6:19–21 TLB

It's very time consuming to deal continually with emergencies
and urgencies in life. It leaves you no time to do what's really important. If you're serious about making your life better and building a
foundation for eternity, simply do what you know you are supposed
to do. That, in a nutshell, is your mission. Mission work is everything you do to move yourself and the world forward—the inspira-
tional, the uplifting, the empowering, and the constructive.
Carrying out your mission is responding to life's possibilities rather
than reacting to life's problems. This mind-set and lifestyle pay huge
dividends forever.

If you are a mother, that's your mission. It's the work God has
given you to do. It's also the blessing God has given you to enjoy. It
is very easy to become so bogged down with the daily details of
motherhood that you miss the blessings.

Managing Your Time to Accomplish More

Some people are list people. They make lists of everything they have
to do and then cross things off as they accomplish them. This makes
them feel good. If they do something that isn't on the list, they write
it down and then cross it off! If they don't finish everything that's on
the list, they move the unfinished items to the next day's list. That
relieves pressure. This is a system that works for many. But there's a
better way to accomplish much and relieve pressure: not only have
a list, but prioritize it.

Not everything has to be done *today*. Figure out what needs to be done right away and what could wait a day or two. Instead of making a list each day, make a weekly list, giving yourself some leeway about which day you're going to do which things. Not everything carries the same weight of importance.

Some things are routine on a daily basis. Obviously you cannot put off making your seven-year-old's school lunch until tomorrow. Having systems in place for accomplishing routine daily tasks is crucial for a well-run household. It provides stability for the family and keeps you sane and less stressed.

Some things are routine on a weekly basis. Schedule laundry and weekly dusting and vacuuming around other chores. I know one mother who dusts and vacuums one room of her five-room house each day so that she doesn't have to do housework on the weekends. The entire house does eventually get cleaned, just one room at a time.

Some things are routine on a seasonal basis. If you live where winters are cold and full of snow, you'll have chores to accomplish twice a year, such as taking out the winter clothes and putting away the summer ones, and then reversing the order in the spring. If you allot two half-days a year for this semiannual ritual, you don't have to think about it for six months.

If you have a husband and children, have a planning session with them. List the things that must be done on a daily basis and assign age-appropriate tasks to everyone in your family. Even the smallest toddler can learn to throw his or her used paper napkin in the wastebasket. You do not have to do every single little thing yourself!

Help by God

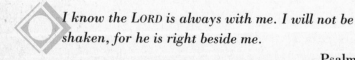

I know the LORD is always with me. I will not be shaken, for he is right beside me.

Psalm 16:8

There are many books on the market full of wonderful suggestions, strategies, and down-to-earth practical solutions to just about any problem a mother will encounter. While you're knee-deep in laundry with one toddler pulling the pots and pans out of the cupboard and a newborn under one arm, it's easy to give up hope that it will ever end! That's the exact time you need to remind yourself that you are a Home Manager, not a slave, and you need to take charge and *manage*. As a Home Manager (or Domestic Engineer, if you like that title better!), your office never closes and your in-box is always full. Someone always wants or needs something all the time. The goal is to organize your life, as it is *now*, to minimize your stress load. That *can* be done!

Organize to Economize

Planning and thinking ahead will help you achieve more in less time. You'll spend less time on routine tasks. You won't be duplicating your efforts as often. You'll feel on top of circumstances instead of under them. Getting organized is the first step in managing your time and, therefore, your life. At least one of the ideas that follow should help you.

Try a personal organizer or planner. This could be a calendar on which you write all the appointments you need to remember, as well as the children's games you want to attend, the social engagements that you have to drive them to, and other places you have to be at a certain time. Write entries on your planner in pencil, not ink! Or purchase a write-on / wipe-off (dry erase) board and color-code each person's schedule: red for one child, green for the new baby, blue for you, purple for your husband, and so forth.

If your life is too complicated for one calendar, read on.

Try daily to-do lists. One of the good things about this method is that you can transfer only the information you need for that day from the larger calendar. Another benefit is that you get a clean slate each day! That keeps you from feeling that you haven't accomplished all you wanted. It should take you only several minutes to transfer the information, and then you have just the one sheet to handle.

Try a weekly plan. A grid with seven vertical columns is the best way to see what the week holds. Label each one with the day of the week and the date.

Try monthly lists. The simplest way to do this is to give each day of the month one line only. Use your own shorthand if necessary to condense the information for any day that has too much for one line.

Try a yearly planner. This is not for details, but rather to give you a quick overview of your long-range plans. Keep the entries general, such as school vacation, family trip, holiday, medical appointments, and so on. Save the details for the daily to-do lists.

Some people also find a zipper bag helpful for holding schedules of school events, transportation such as trains and buses, game times, coupons, and doctor appointment cards with times and phone numbers on them.

It's also helpful to have a portable file of phone numbers and addresses for repair and maintenance people you frequently call, as well as doctors, dentists, and other health providers. It beats carrying the phone book around with you!

Having all this information at your fingertips and in one place, whether you are away from the house or at home, is so convenient that you'll wonder how you ever got along without using a planner/organizer!

Know What Works for You (As Well As What Doesn't)

What works for someone else might not work for you. Only you can decide what methods and strategies mesh with your schedule, your family, and your own goals for managing your time. Ask yourself what you're trying to accomplish (the goal), what time frame you have to accomplish it in (the deadline), and how much of a hurry you're in to accomplish it (the priority). You can do this for every area of your life: home, work, family, children, marriage, and yourself. From your answers, you'll detect a pattern and get some direction.

Develop a Routine and Follow It

Some people get up in the morning with no idea of what they're going to do that day. (You should be so lucky, right?) They cope with whatever comes up as it comes up. They don't plan; they react. If you're bouncing back from pregnancy, you cannot afford to do that!

If babies need routine, new moms need it more! Your newborn will have needs you'll have to anticipate and plan for. Your body will demand your attention as well, especially if you truly want to get back to your prepregnancy weight. Having a daily routine for your baby is of prime importance, of course, since giving him or her the right start in life is your responsibility. A routine helps both you and your baby feel comfortable and safe. It also makes it easier to remember things that need to be done and, ultimately, it saves precious time that you would spend just reacting to things as they come up or doing them as they occur to you.

Prepare for the Next Day Before Going to Bed

If the lunches are prepared and in the refrigerator, the clothes are ready to put on, and the car has enough gas to get all the family members where they're going first thing in the morning, you'll get a better night's sleep and your morning will not be as hectic. You'll start the day *ahead*, not behind.

Organize Your Space So You Don't Spend Time Looking for Things

Whether it's a closet, a kitchen drawer, or your office, having things in predictable spots where you can see them and get what you need saves hundreds of hours a year. If you've ever had to delay your departure because everyone had to stop and help you look for your car keys, you know I'm telling the truth!

Organize Your Closets by Outfits That Go Together So You Don't Spend Time Trying to Decide What to Wear

This may sound like overkill, but it truly does save time. If you have six tops that go with six bottoms and they all coordinate with each other, life is just easier. Time spent staring at a disorganized closet is not only discouraging, but also a huge time waster.

Mend or Repair Clothing or Accessories As Soon As Possible

If you cannot mend things right away, put them in a basket or some other container and schedule an hour in front of the television or the fireplace to take care of them. Putting unrepaired clothing back into the drawer or closet is another time waster because you will put them on, then have to change. Sewing on buttons in front of a cozy fire on a chilly evening with a mug of herbal tea may sound like a mini-vacation to you!

Invest One Hour a Week to Plan the Next Week

You can plan the upcoming week in half an hour if you are using some of the organizing and planning tips we've already discussed. It will be time well invested, because your mind will be ready to relax by Friday or Saturday night, and you won't have to wonder what you've forgotten that's going to hit you first thing Monday morning. Planning is a great stress reducer.

Delegate

I've mentioned that you don't have to do everything around the house, and you shouldn't. Even the smallest child can learn to do household chores that are at his or her level of coping skills. If you're delegating to children, be patient with them while they're learning how you want things done. If you have teenagers, ask them to plan and serve dinner one night a week and clean up the kitchen afterward. (Your husband could do that too!)

If you do everything for your family, how will they ever learn how to handle responsibility? Part of your job is to grow them into responsible adulthood. Start now, if you haven't already. One word of advice: if they're cooking dinner, stay out of the kitchen. Pour some bubble bath into the tub or take a long, relaxing shower. This should be free time for you, so enjoy it!

Learn to Say No

Saying no doesn't mean you're a bad person. It means you have your priorities straight. Those priorities are God, family, and yourself—in that order. It's been said that *no* is the only word needed for good time management. Examine why you always say *yes* to people who put demands on your time. Make sure it's not because you feel you wouldn't be as good a mother if you say no occasionally—or as good a friend or neighbor. When people ask you to do something, it's not a command. You have the choice of responding one of three ways: yes, no, or "Not right now . . . let me pray about it." Exercise your freedom of choice and say no to requests that do not advance your goals or contribute to the things that are most important to you (your values).

Don't Put It Down; Put It Away

That goes for you as well as your children. Why handle something twice when you could handle it only once and be done with it? Teaching your children to put things away breeds responsibility and eliminates 90 percent of the picking up after people that usually comes with being a mom. It's a great time-saver.

Train Older Children to Wash and Dress the Little Ones

At the beginning, this will take some time investment on your part. Help the older ones at first to be sure they understand how you want things done. Make it a game for the little ones, and they'll soon adjust to having their big brother or sister help them.

Leave the Kitchen Ready for Morning Before You Go to Bed Every Night

Having a tidy kitchen to walk into first thing in the morning starts the day off right—with a sense of calm and orderliness. It really doesn't take long to do the dishes the night before (or run the dishwasher), wipe the counters, clean the stovetop, and put things away. What greets your eyes first thing in the morning can make a huge difference in the tone of your day.

Face Problems

Don't ignore them. (They rarely go away on their own.)

Do Two Things at the Same Time

This is called *synchronization* or *multitasking*. You probably already do some of this: picking up the dry cleaning on the way to the grocery store so you don't have to make two separate trips, for example. You can also prepare dinner while you do laundry. You can iron shirts while you supervise your children's homework session. You can work out while you talk to a friend on the phone. (I do that routinely.)

Be Prepared for Unexpected Circumstances

Life is full of surprises. Keep both the diaper bag and snack bags stocked and ready. You never know when you'll have to leave the house quickly, and if you have to stop to prepare these two necessary bags, you'll wish you had replenished them when you had the time. Being prepared always saves you time and stress.

Buy Foods in Bulk

It also saves time to buy foods in bulk whenever possible. When the grocery store has a buy-one-get-one-free sale, stock up. You save shopping time, cooking time, and preparation time. You also eliminate stress. Your family comes home to a peaceful home where everything is under control. Even your baby picks up on the difference between stress and calm.

Cook More Than One Meal at a Time

For your own peace of mind, when you've had a hectic day and aren't feeling well, it's a wonderful feeling to know that you've got dinner covered. Cook double-dinners (enough for two nights), and freeze what you don't eat the first night. You'll appreciate it some night the next week.

Invest in Oven Bags

These little plastic wonders allow you to cook a roast with the vegetables to perfection. They also allow you to give yourself a second night off from cooking by serving the leftovers on another night.

Do Not Make Your Children's Beds, and Teach Them to Clean Their Own Rooms

You're not doing your children any favors when you make their beds for them after they're old enough to learn to do it themselves. Teach them how to do it, and insist that they do. Never mind what it looks like at first; they'll improve if you coach them. (Their future spouses will thank you for your efforts someday!)

Shop When the Stores Are Less Busy

It will take less time if you're not battling the crowds. I find the best times are early in the morning or late at night. If that doesn't work for you, even mid-morning and mid-afternoon are better than peak times (just before mealtimes).

Shop with a List and Avoid Impulse Buying

This takes discipline. Keep a running list at home, and make everyone responsible for writing down what he or she needs. Make this a house rule: If you see that you're running out of an item, put it on the list. (I don't know about you, but I absolutely hate running out of something when I think I've got plenty.) You can take the list one step further and have three columns: *Item Name, Out,* and *Low.* Whoever writes the item on the list under *Item Name* puts a check mark under either *Out* or *Low.*

Don't Take the Children Grocery Shopping with You

You can shop faster and stick to your list better when you're alone. The exception would be a teenager whom you're teaching how to shop. That's best done with either one or two teens. After that it turns into a party and a hunt for the cutest bag boy.

For Moms Who Work at Home

Working at home is a double-sided coin. Your baby will cooperate most of the time by following the routine you have established for feeding and napping. It's fairly easy to adjust your work schedule around a newborn or infant.

Working at home is a privilege many women envy. There are good and bad things about it, though. Most mothers who work at home say the good outweighs the bad. For example, you can work in your bunny slippers if you want to, but your toddlers will think you're home to play with *them.* It takes patience, repetitive training, and planning activities for them so you can actually get some work accomplished. You'll have to train your older children that when you are working, they need to think of you as being at the office and give you some time and space. Eventually your family will adjust to your work schedule and honor it.

If you notice that your children are interrupting you frequently despite reminders that you need to finish the work you're doing, try scheduling some time with each of your children where it's just the two of you. Or, if that simply doesn't work, consider hiring someone to come in and watch them for a few hours each day while you work.

For Moms Who Work Outside the Home

If you are a mother and also work outside of the home, you are doing double duty, sometimes referred to as *double-daying,* because you spend the equivalent of two whole days doing two full-time jobs in a twenty-four-hour period. Trying to find time for yourself is an even bigger challenge for you than for the mothers who work at home.

When you get home from work and all you want to do is kick off your shoes and put your feet up, you can't. There's dinner to prepare, the children who want your attention, and a husband who is also tired from working all day and wants to spend time with you. And then there's the dog that is bored from being alone all day and looks to you for nurturing as well!

Go ahead and kick off those shoes, and put your feet up for five glorious minutes. Let your family know that's what you're doing, and tell them if they want you to be a fun companion the rest of the evening, you need that time to yourself.

 One Mom Finds the Time for Herself

All her life, Darcy really loved to read. As a child, she read to escape a not-too-happy home life. As a teenager, she read romance novels and dreamed of what her married life would be like. After graduation, she landed a great job that she really loved and because of that she read everything she could to help her get ahead in her career. As a newlywed, she devoured books on homemaking and making relationships work. As a new mother, however, she found precious little time to read anything except food labels and baby books! When the baby was six weeks old, Darcy returned to work because she had to: her husband was in the National Guard and had been called to active duty.

After work, Darcy picked up the baby from day care, went home to an empty house, and began preparing dinner. All she really wanted to do was curl up with a good book that would take her away from what her life had become: all work and no time for herself. It's not that she didn't love her baby; she did—more than she thought was possible. She was just so stressed and tired! Clearly she had to do something about the situation. But what?

The thing she missed the most was reading for pleasure. Remembering that she was frequently standing in line or caught in rush-hour traffic, Darcy realized she could probably find an hour a day for reading if she grabbed the opportunities in bits and pieces. Five minutes in the line at the bank, twenty minutes in the doctor's waiting room, fifteen minutes over lunch—it all added up. She began carrying a book with her wherever she went.

That definitely helped, but there was still that awkward time after she arrived at home after work, when the baby needed her attention and she needed to prepare dinner. She needed a halfway house! Or maybe the house was the wrong place to refresh herself before tackling the home responsibilities.

One evening Darcy decided to take the baby for a walk before getting dinner and starting the other chores. It didn't matter if dinner was at 6 PM instead of 5:30. She quickly changed into a jogging outfit and her sneakers, bundled the baby into a snuggly sling, and headed out the door. She walked fifteen minutes away from home, then turned around and walked back. Both she and the baby had a great time, and she was able to take on her home responsibilities without resentment—because she had found a way to do something for herself. The time together was good for both of them, and it gave Darcy the break she needed between work and home.

▲ ▲ ▲

Make Time for Yourself

Whether you are a stay-at-home mother, you run a business from your home, or you go to work outside the home, finding time for yourself is a real problem. It's also a necessity if you are to enjoy motherhood to the fullest. If you don't take care of you, who will?

Here are some ideas on finding those mini-breaks in your day that will revive and refresh you.

Exercise

If you exercise for 30-40 minutes a day, you will see tremendous changes in your body, your soul, and your spirit. You're probably thinking you don't have a half-hour to spend on yourself! Yes, you do! You just need to rearrange a few things—such as what time you get up.

Actually, a half-hour of exercise will end up saving you time, because you'll be so energized and feel so good afterward that you'll accomplish more in less time. Your mind will work better, problems will take on the correct perspective instead of looming like giants, and your confidence level will increase. You can have great talks with God while you're exercising, even if it's "God, please help me up this next hill!" (He will.) You'll be ready to take on the world!

Exercise is an incredible boost for your ability to cope. It does wonderful things for your overall health, too, so you'll feel better physically, mentally, and spiritually. What's not to love about exercise? And why aren't you doing it? (See pages 135 to 208 for ideas.)

Decrease Your Load

If you delegate some of your responsibilities to others, you'll gain some time that could be used for exercising or some other activity you enjoy. You don't really have to do it all; you just have to make sure it all gets done. I know I've touched on this already, but it bears repeating.

Never Go Anywhere Without a Book, a Tape, or a Project

Time spent sitting in traffic or waiting in line can be mini-vacations for your brain if you have a means of escape handy. Even a few minutes refreshes your mind and your spirit. Turning waiting in doctors' offices into time for you requires an attitude adjustment, but you can do it by carrying a book, a tape, needlepoint, or some other small portable craft project with you.

Turn Errand Time into a Fun Experience

When you have half a dozen errands to do on one trip, include a *refresh stop* for yourself at a coffee shop. Order a cup of herbal tea, and just savor the time alone. Don't think about anything on your to-do list. You'll emerge ready to finish your errands in good time.

Learn to Meditate

Meditation is incredibly relaxing and gets your mind on something other than your hectic life. Many books tell how to develop meditation skills, but the simplest instruction is this: Empty your mind of everything except the one concept on which you've chosen to meditate. Spend fifteen minutes in a quiet place where you will not be interrupted and concentrate on this thing in all its facets.

For example, think of one characteristic of God: His faithfulness to you. How many times He has met your needs. How He has always been available to you. How He has answered all your prayers—maybe yes, maybe no, maybe "Wait awhile," but He answered. Think about how great He is and how there are no words big enough to describe Him and not enough time to thank Him for all He's done for you.

I guarantee you that if you can spend at least five minutes meditating on God in this way, it will change your life. Of course, you can meditate about other things as well. But this is especially helpful to me, and I think it will be to you too.

Clean the Bathroom

(No, this isn't in the wrong place!) Tell the family you're going to clean the bathroom; it will take an hour, and you're going to do it alone. Do the cleaning first. Then light candles, put on some music, fill the tub with a hot bubble bath, and indulge yourself in a good book. True escape!

Write in Your Journal for at Least Fifteen Minutes

Journaling is a wonderful escape. It doesn't take long, and it is very beneficial. It lets you express your thoughts, verbalize your dreams, voice your cares, and it's private! After a month of journaling, go back and read the entries. You'll gain knowledge of yourself and insights into areas that need working on.

Turn on Some Music and Dance with the Baby
After Everyone Has Left for the Day

You'll both love it!

Write a Letter (Not an E-Mail) to a Friend

E-mail has just about obliterated the fine art of letter writing. Splurge on some gorgeous stationery and a nice pen, and write to someone who will appreciate getting a special letter in the mail. Speak from your heart. Mention good times you had together. This means a great deal to older people especially, such as a relative or neighbor you no longer live near. You'll feel good for being so thoughtful, and you'll spread the blessing to the recipient of your letter.

Take a Class or Attend a Special-Interest Group
(Such As a Bible-Study Class)

Meeting with people who have the same interests as you is a great way to give yourself a break.

Schedule a Massage with a Licensed Therapist,
or Spend a Half-Day at a Spa

Obviously, this will require planning and take more than a few minutes. But it is worth it, even if you only get to do it once a month.

Spend an Hour at a Museum or Art Gallery

Nothing gets you out of yourself like seeing what others have done or are doing to bring beauty and interest to the world around you.

Let the Answering Machine Get the Phone

If you allow it, the people who call you can eat huge holes in your day and cause more stress by putting you behind schedule. You have to be firm with well-meaning friends who want to talk for hours when you do not have time. By choosing your words carefully, you can solve the problem without offending anyone: "I'd love to talk, but right now I'm late for something. Could I call you tomorrow morning at 9:30?" This lets the friend know you want to talk, but you have a responsibility you must tend to right then.

Saying you are late for something is noncommittal. It doesn't mean you have a doctor's appointment. It means you have some responsibility you must meet. It could be your time with God; it could be your walk with the dog; it could be your time set aside for yourself; it could be another friend or your child who needs your help. These are all responsibilities you have accepted and committed to, and you need to fulfill them. So you are not misleading your phone friend by saying that.

Do not let others unintentionally rob you of your ability to control your own time. On the other hand, do follow through on your commitment to call your friend back at 9:30 the next morning, or you'll have to spend even more time apologizing to her!

Interruptions by God

It takes no effort at all for someone or something to mess up your neat little to-do list. Of course, not every interruption is from God! So you need to pray over your list and your responses to life's interruptions as well. A neighbor knocks on your door. Her car battery is dead and she needs to get to a doctor's appointment. Could you take her? Your mother calls. She fell and broke her wrist and will need help for the next few weeks with household chores. Your husband calls and has to go out of town on a short business trip. Could you do the laundry today instead of waiting until Friday? (I know what you're thinking: *I'm lucky he called!*)

We've all been there, and we all know what happens to our careful planning and detailed lists. But this is life—ever changing, ever challenging, ever interesting, ever stimulating, ever demanding, and ever rewarding when you learn to take it as it comes. God is not surprised at any of life's emergency situations and daily disasters. He knew they were going to hit, and He's ready to go through them with you.

Maybe some of the things on your to-do list are not things He had for you to do today at all. That's the tricky thing about lists: you cannot be possessive about them. Give your list to God, and allow Him to arrange your days. You'll get the important things accomplished. The rest can wait. That might not be your neighbor knocking on your door; it might be God, giving you an opportunity to be His hands and feet by helping someone in need.

Setting Goals

Now that we've moved beyond crisis management, let me ask you something: What are your dreams? What would you like to accomplish in your life? A goal is one step beyond a dream. A goal is a dream with feet.

You can (and should) set goals in every area of your life: spiritual, personal, educational, physical, financial, relational, and occupational. If you're going to achieve your goals, you'll need to apply the principles of time management we've been discussing, and you'll need to seek God's wisdom in setting goals that honor Him, are consistent with your values, and are achievable. (You don't just get up one morning and say, "I think I'll learn to pilot a plane today." Not only does that take planning and organization, it takes time and money. You need to set realistic goals and give yourself time to achieve them.)

The Skinny on Time Management

I can summarize effective time management in five terms: goal setting, prioritizing, planning, scheduling, and rewarding.

Goal setting is deciding what is important to you and when you would like to achieve it. Suppose you live in Minnesota and you want to escape the snow and ice in early March. You'd like to go somewhere warm and toast in the sun for a week. Brazil has always intrigued you. You set the goal of spending the second week in March somewhere in Brazil—you don't care where, as long as it's warm!

Prioritizing is determining what needs to be done in what order so that you can reach your goals. You make a list of everything that you have to do to step off the plane and feel that moist, warm breeze ruffle your hair on the ninth of March, which is ten months away. On the first list you simply write things down as they occur to you: get a haircut, lose twenty pounds, get a new bathing suit, learn Portuguese, buy the plane ticket, research resorts and hotels, get brochures from a travel agent, search the Internet for information on South America, save the money to pay for the trip.

Obviously these are in no particular order. You cannot get off the plane before you save the money to pay for the ticket! So you make a second list from the first, putting the things in proper order. You will accomplish several things at the same time, for example, saving the money for the trip and losing twenty pounds. But you're *good* at multitasking, right?

Planning is how you are going to achieve the steps you need to take to arrive at each of your goals. How are you going to save the money for the trip? Should you get a second job? Sock money away from the grocery money? Sell some furniture? How are you going to lose twenty pounds in ten months? Give up ice cream? Add more Food by God to your daily diet? Exercise regularly?

Scheduling is putting together a time frame for working your plan. To get the best airfare you need to book your trip three months in advance, by the end of December. Hmmm . . . that would make a nice Christmas present for yourself! That means you must save the money for the trip over the next seven months. How much money do you need to have by December, and how much can you save for the incidentals between December and your departure date? But wait! First you need to find out how much the entire trip is going to cost. You'll need to do some research in the next two weeks in order to figure that out. But it will be so much fun planning it all!

Rewarding is taking the time to reward the achievement of your goals. You achieve every major goal by meeting a series of mini-goals contained within that goal. You don't have to wait until you actually achieve the large end-goal of stepping off the plane in Rio de Janeiro to reward yourself. When you save enough money to pay for the plane ticket, why not reward yourself by attending a lecture on South American culture? When you weigh in at twenty pounds less than you did the day you set the goal of losing it, why not reward yourself by buying that new bathing suit you want to take with you to Rio? Of course, the biggest reward will be arriving at your destination and realizing you did it: you set a huge goal and you made it happen! Give yourself a pat on the back for me. I'm proud of you.

25 | Scheduling a Better Family Life

Once you get your time under control, you will have enough for everything you are supposed to do, as well as some very important fun things. Here are some ways to improve your family life and cement family relationships.

Have a Family Devotional Time

Many books are available to help you with a structured devotional time. The basic elements are a short Bible verse or passage, an explanation of the same, and a time of prayer. Children should be encouraged to ask questions, voice opinions and concerns, make prayer requests, and pray aloud. None of this has to be scary for anyone. If you've never had a family devotional time, start slowly, but start. It will pay eternal dividends in your family life, both corporately and individually. It's not just a nice saying that *the family that prays together, stays together.*

Invite Your Husband Out on a Date

Whether it's spur-of-the-moment or planned several days in advance, everyone likes to be considered special enough to be invited out on a date by the person he or she loves. Having a baby puts restraints on a relationship. Your husband needs to know that you want to spend quality time with him alone, without the baby (or the other children). Hire a sitter, get your hair done, and go for it!

Spend Some Time One-on-One with Each of Your Children Every Day

Don't forget that they are adjusting to the new baby in their lives too. They need to feel that they are as important to you as the new addition to the family. With younger children, turn off the television and get out the crayons and coloring books and work on adjoining pages together. Reading together is always a good idea for some quality time. With older children, go for a walk or a short ride in the car. Use this time to find out what's going on in their lives and see how they're feeling about the changes in the family. Communication is key to preventing potential problems.

Spend Time with Your Family at Home in the Evening

Play games or read a book together and then discuss it. This teaches the children to be content with the simple pleasures of life and to value and enjoy their home life. It will mean a lot to them later—through memories, and through principles they pass on to their own children. It sets in concrete some very important family values.

Remember Your Family Is Just That: Your Family

Don't compare it to other people's families. You are a unique unit. God has put your family together for a purpose: to love and help each other through life, and to give honor to Him. Each family is different from all the others. Revel in your uniqueness.

Be Flexible

In *Fiddler on the Roof,* during a serious discussion with God about tradition and flexibility, the hero says, "If I don't bend, I'll break." That applies to being too rigid on things that don't matter much in the long run. For example, if you're trying to train your children to hang up the towels instead of leaving them on the floor, how much does it really matter if they are hanging a little bit crooked? At least they're on the towel rod!

Sometimes, in our search for validation as excellent mothers, we expect too much from those who are unable to give it. The other danger is to expect too little from those who aren't even trying. Flexibility also helps when your plans are pushed aside for someone else's idea or an emergency. Life is give-and-take. The goal is some give and some take on everyone's part. Flexibility takes the pressure off you, and everyone else.

When You Take the Dog for a Walk, Take the Children Too

Not many activities are both great relaxers and energizers at the same time, but walking definitely is one of them. Make walking the dog a special family time, even for the dog. Anything you can do as a family is good.

Slow Down

Life is not an Olympic event. Learn to savor every moment. One way to slow down quickly is to simply close your eyes (unless you're driving!), and count backwards from one hundred, one count per deep breath. This has a very calming influence on your body, your soul, and your spirit. It works on children, too, if they're old enough to know how to count backwards.

Don't Go to Every Available Meeting

Networking is vital if you are in business. Support groups are vital when you're a new mom. Spending time with others in the same boat as you is called *fellowship* (two fellows in the same ship). All of this is important and helpful. But at some point, meetings and gatherings will cross the line and begin to take over your life if you attend too many. You do not have to be at *every* meeting. Don't over-commit your time to things that do not help you achieve your goals and keep your priorities straight. Set limits on the number of meetings, coffees, and playgroups you attend. Too much of a good thing is not good.

Life by God

God has a plan for your life, and it's a good one. You don't want to miss any of it! (Even the stuff that's on your to-do lists!) He wants you to be healthy, happy, peaceful, and wise. You can do that while enjoying the process if you continually give your life back to God (who gave it to you in the first place). Nothing will make Him happier!

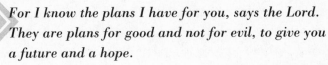

For I know the plans I have for you, says the Lord. They are plans for good and not for evil, to give you a future and a hope.

—Jeremiah 29:11 TLB

 Keeping Priorities in Order

In the book of Acts, chapter nine, we meet someone who was a wonder woman, if ever there was one: Dorcas. The motivating principle of this woman's life was love—love for God, which continually expressed itself in doing good for others, even those she did not know. Love got her out of bed in the morning and kept her fingers flying all day long. Love wore out her sandals as she went from low-income housing development to local jail to nursing home and finally to soup kitchen. Interestingly, her name means gazelle. Can't you just envision her, gracefully leaping from one good deed to another, spreading joy everywhere she went? Quick and graceful, that was Dorcas.

We don't know when she first . . . made God the center of her life, but we do know that she loved him and embraced the Gospel with all her strength. Dorcas wasn't one to do things halfway! When she worked, she gave it everything she had, holding nothing back—living each moment to the hilt. If this woman had had a nickname, it should have been *Alka-Seltzer.* The gratitude and love for God just bubbled up deep inside Dorcas' spirit and effervesced all over those she came in contact with. She neither planned to be that way, nor could she help it.

It wasn't possible to keep all that love inside, so she became a one-woman

Salvation Army. Benevolent, compassionate, and generous beyond the norm, Dorcas gave so generously of her time, her talents, and her money, that 2,000 years later, her name is still synonymous with gracious giving to those in need. Many churches have their Dorcas Societies—groups where the women do all they can to alleviate the situations of those in their communities who are in physical need. Often they collect used clothes, clean and mend them, and deliver them to those who need them. It's not unusual for a Dorcas Society to prepare entire layettes for unwed mothers of newborns one week, and knit or crochet lap robes for the local nursing home residents the next week. Because Dorcas held nothing back from God, thousands of lives have been blessed for thousands of years. We don't know if she had any children, or even if she was married. But what a legacy she left you and me!

From Dorcas we learn the formula for true joy in life. It's a simple one: God first, others next, yourself last . . . If you keep your priorities in this order, you will be deeply, truly, unshakably, effervescently happy.*

*Alice Hellstrom Anderson, Through the Bible in High Heels (Belleville, Ont., Canada: Guardian Books, 2002), 118–119. Used by permission.

▲ ▲ ▲

The key to enjoying your Life by God—and coping with all it brings—is twofold: surrender and flexibility. Make your lists and make your plans, but surrender your will to His and let Him alter your plans and order your days. Don't get married to your to-do list. Don't think the only good home is one that is clean enough to eat off the floor. Don't lose sight of what's really important in life: love, health, providing for your family's needs and taking care of yourself so you can do all of that with excellence.

Just as pregnancy is an individualized experience, so is bouncing back from pregnancy. God made you and your Body by God unique and then threw away the mold! That's totally amazing to me. He not only made you, He holds your body, soul, and spirit in the palm of His hand as you bounce back from the birth of your child.

It's been a good experience for me to write this book, and what has helped me the most is my deep desire to help other women learn how to make their pregnancies easier and healthier, as well as their bouncing back both a fulfilling and fun time in their lives. If I did it, so can you!

I would love to hear from you! How has this book helped you? What changes have you made in your life that might be of help to others? Tell me your stories by writing to me at:

Dr. Sheri Lerner
604 Front St.
Celebration, FL 34747

or e-mailing me at:

DrSheri@TheBodyByGod.com

If you would like more information about chiropractic or Dr. Sheri's clinic, call 321-939-2328.

Charts and Forms

The following charts are from Ben Lerner's *Body by God: The Owner's Manual for Maximized Living,* also from Nelson Books, a Division of Thomas Nelson Publishers. Used by permission.

Personal BBG 40-Day Plan Playbook

MONDAY

Time:	Time:	Time:	Time:	Time:	Time:	Time:	Time:	Time:
Life:	Life:	Life:	Life:	Life:	Life:	Life:	Life:	Life:
Missionary Work:	Missionary Work:	Missionary Work:	Missionary Work:	Missionary Work:	Missionary Work:	Missionary Work:	Missionary Work:	Missionary Work:
Special Time:	Special Time:	Special Time:	Special Time:	Special Time:	Special Time:	Special Time:	Special Time:	Special Time:
(SYL)	(SYL)	(SYL)	(SYL)	(SYL)	(SYL)	(SYL)	(SYL)	(SYL)

SOLID YELLOW LINE (SYL)

TUESDAY

Time:	Time:	Time:	Time:	Time:	Time:	Time:	Time:	Time:
Life:	Life:	Life:	Life:	Life:	Life:	Life:	Life:	Life:
Missionary Work:	Missionary Work:	Missionary Work:	Missionary Work:	Missionary Work:	Missionary Work:	Missionary Work:	Missionary Work:	Missionary Work:
Special Time:	Special Time:	Special Time:	Special Time:	Special Time:	Special Time:	Special Time:	Special Time:	Special Time:
(SYL)	(SYL)	(SYL)	(SYL)	(SYL)	(SYL)	(SYL)	(SYL)	(SYL)

SOLID YELLOW LINE (SYL)

Personal BBG 40-Day Plan Playbook

WEDNESDAY

Time:	Time:	Time:	Time:	Time:	Time:	Time:	Time:
Life:	Life:	Life:	Life:	Life:	Life:	Life:	Life:
Missionary Work:	Missionary Work:	Missionary Work:	Missionary Work:	Missionary Work:	Missionary Work:	Missionary Work:	Missionary Work:
Special Time:	Special Time:	Special Time:	Special Time:	Special Time:	Special Time:	Special Time:	Special Time:
(SYL)	(SYL)	(SYL)	(SYL)	(SYL)	(SYL)	(SYL)	(SYL)

SOLID YELLOW LINE (SYL)

THURSDAY

Time:	Time:	Time:	Time:	Time:	Time:	Time:	Time:
Life:	Life:	Life:	Life:	Life:	Life:	Life:	Life:
Missionary Work:	Missionary Work:	Missionary Work:	Missionary Work:	Missionary Work:	Missionary Work:	Missionary Work:	Missionary Work:
Special Time:	Special Time:	Special Time:	Special Time:	Special Time:	Special Time:	Special Time:	Special Time:
(SYL)	(SYL)	(SYL)	(SYL)	(SYL)	(SYL)	(SYL)	(SYL)

SOLID YELLOW LINE (SYL)

Personal BBG 40-Day Plan Playbook

FRIDAY

Time:	Time:	Time:	Time:	Time:	Time:	Time:	Time:
Life:	Life:	Life:	Life:	Life:	Life:	Life:	Life:
Missionary Work:	Missionary Work:	Missionary Work:	Missionary Work:	Missionary Work:	Missionary Work:	Missionary Work:	Missionary Work:
Special Time:	Special Time:	Special Time:	Special Time:	Special Time:	Special Time:	Special Time:	Special Time:
(SYL)	(SYL)	(SYL)	(SYL)	(SYL)	(SYL)	(SYL)	(SYL)

SOLID YELLOW LINE (SYL)

SATURDAY

Time:	Time:	Time:	Time:	Time:	Time:	Time:	Time:
Life:	Life:	Life:	Life:	Life:	Life:	Life:	Life:
Missionary Work:	Missionary Work:	Missionary Work:	Missionary Work:	Missionary Work:	Missionary Work:	Missionary Work:	Missionary Work:
Special Time:	Special Time:	Special Time:	Special Time:	Special Time:	Special Time:	Special Time:	Special Time:
(SYL)	(SYL)	(SYL)	(SYL)	(SYL)	(SYL)	(SYL)	(SYL)

SOLID YELLOW LINE (SYL)

Personal BBG 40-Day Plan Playbook

SUNDAY

Time:	Time:	Time:	Time:	Time:	Time:	Time:	Time:
Life:	Life:	Life:	Life:	Life:	Life:	Life:	Life:
Missionary Work:	Missionary Work:	Missionary Work:	Missionary Work:	Missionary Work:	Missionary Work:	Missionary Work:	Missionary Work:
Special Time:	Special Time:	Special Time:	Special Time:	Special Time:	Special Time:	Special Time:	Special Time:
(SYL)	(SYL)	(SYL)	(SYL)	(SYL)	(SYL)	(SYL)	(SYL)

SOLID YELLOW LINE (SYL)

MORNING | BODY BY GOD UN-DIET | Nutrient Evaluation Form

Date	Real Time	Intended Time by God
	_____ A.M./P.M.	_____ A.M./P.M.

Actual Food	Why You Ate/Drank?	Planned Food by God
Carbohydrate:		Carbohydrate:
Protein:		Protein:
Fat:		Fat:
Liquid:		Liquid:
Food by Man:		Food by Man:
How you felt after eating	How you felt 1-2 hours later	

MIDDAY   BODY BY GOD UN-DIET   Nutrient Evaluation Form

Date	Real Time	Intended Time by God
	_____ A.M./P.M.	_____ A.M./P.M.

Actual Food	Why You Ate/Drank?	Planned Food by God
Carbohydrate:		Carbohydrate:
Protein:		Protein:
Fat:		Fat:
Liquid:		Liquid:
Food by Man:		Food by Man:
How you felt after eating	How you felt 1-2 hours later	

EVENING | BODY BY GOD UN-DIET | Nutrient Evaluation Form

Date	Real Time	Intended Time by God
	_____ A.M./P.M.	_____ A.M./P.M.

Actual Food | Why You Ate/Drank? | Planned Food by God

Actual Food

Carbohydrate:

Protein:

Fat:

Liquid:

Food by Man:

How you felt after eating

Planned Food by God

Carbohydrate:

Protein:

Fat:

Liquid:

Food by Man:

How you felt 1-2 hours later

PERSONAL AEROBIC ROUTINES

30-MINUTE CARDIOVASCULAR MOVEMENT
(+10 MINUTE WARM-UP/COOLDOWN = 40 MINUTE TOTAL)

FOR FAT BURNING

Name: _____
Age: _____ Gender: _____
ACTIVITY: _____

FUR - Fat-Utilization Rate   PER - Performance Enhancement Rate   SUR - Sugar-Utilization Rate

FUR: _____   PER: _____   SUR: _____

| MOVING ZONE LEVELS | | | | |
TIME (Elapsed)	TIME (Per Stage)	HEART RATE	SPEED/INCLINE OR LEVEL/RPM	HEART RATE (Real)
0:00	0:00	Resting Heart Rate (RHR)+	Mph/	RHR
5:00	5:00	Below - FUR	Mph/	
7:00	2:00	Near - FUR	Mph/	
9:00	2:00	Nearer - FUR	Mph/	
14:00	5:00	First 1% - FUR	Mph/	
19:00	5:00	First 10% - FUR	Mph/	
24:00	5:00	First 50% - FUR	Mph/	
29:00	5:00	First 10% - FUR	Mph/	
32:00	3:00	First 1% - FUR	Mph/	
35:00	3:00	Near - FUR	Mph/	
40:00	5:00	Below - FUR - RHR+	Mph/	

PERSONAL AEROBIC ROUTINES

40-Minute Cardiovascular Movement

(+10 Minute Warm-Up/Cooldown= 50 Minute Total)

FOR FAT BURNING AND IMPROVED PERFORMANCE

Name: _____

Age: _____ Gender: _____

ACTIVITY: _____

WARNING - Before you begin: Never start an exercise program without first consulting your physician. Those with a personal history of heart disease, high blood pressure, high cholesterol, cancer, diabetes, or who smoke or are overweight should begin exercising with professional supervision.

FUR - Fat-Utilization Rate   PER - Performance Enhancement Rate   SUR - Sugar-Utilization Rate

FUR: _____   PER: _____   SUR: _____

| MOVING ZONE LEVELS | | | | |
TIME (Elapsed)	TIME (Per Stage)	HEART RATE	SPEED/INCLINE OR LEVEL/RPM	HEART RATE (Real)
0:00	0:00	Resting Heart Rate (RHR)+	0 Mph/	
5:00	5:00	Below - FUR	Mph/	
7:00	2:00	Near - FUR	Mph/	
9:00	2:00	Nearer - FUR	Mph/	
11:00	2:00	First 1% - FUR	Mph/	
13:00	2:00	First 10% - FUR	Mph/	
15:00	2:00	First 10% - FUR	Mph/	
18:00	3:00	First 50% - FUR	Mph/	
21:00	3:00	Last 50% - FUR	Mph/	
25:00	4:00	First 50% - PER	Mph/	
29:00	4:00	First 50% - PER	Mph/	
33:00	4:00	Last 50% - PER	Mph/	
36:00	3:00	Last 50% - PER	Mph/	
39:00	3:00	PER - FUR	Mph/	
42:00	3:00	Last 50% - FUR	Mph/	
45:00	3:00	First 50% - FUR	Mph/	
50:00	5:00	First 10% - FUR - RHR +	Mph/	

PERSONAL AEROBIC ROUTINES

40-Minute Cardiovascular Movement

(+10 Minute Warm-Up/Cooldown= 50 Minute Total)

FOR FAT BURNING AND SPORTS/PEAK PERFORMANCE

Name: _____

Age: _____ **Gender:** _____

ACTIVITY: _____

FUR - Fat-Utilization Rate   **PER** - Performance Enhancement Rate   **SUR** - Sugar-Utilization Rate

FUR: _____   **PER:** _____   **SUR:** _____

MOVING ZONE LEVELS TIME (Elapsed)	TIME (Per Stage)	HEART RATE	SPEED/INCLINE OR LEVEL/RPM	HEART RATE (Real)
0:00	0:00	Resting Heart Rate+	0 Mph	
5:00	5:00	Below - FUR	Mph	
7:00	2:00	Near - FUR	Mph	
9:00	2:00	Nearer - FUR	Mph	
11:00	2:00	First 1% - FUR	Mph	
13:00	2:00	First 50% - FUR	Mph	
15:00	2:00	First 50% - PER	Mph	
17:00	2:00	SUR	Mph	
19:00	2:00	PER - FUR	Mph	
21:00	2:00	PER	Mph	
24:00	3:00	SUR	Mph	
26:00	2:00	PER - FUR	Mph	
28:00	2:00	PER	Mph	
32:00	4:00	SUR	Mph	
34:00	2:00	PER - FUR	Mph	
36:00	2:00	PER	Mph	
41:00	5:00	SUR	Mph	
45:00	4:00	PER - FUR	Mph	
50:00	5:00	FUR - RHR+	Mph	

The Daily BBG Fitness Program

Body Parts: ....

Real Date	Real Time	Intended Date	Intended Time by God
	.........A.M./P.M.		.........A.M./P.M.

Types of Sets
Legs:
Upper Body:

- Decline - **D**
  15 - 5 reps
  12 - 5 reps

- Pause - **P**
  12 - 0 reps
  12 - 0 reps

- Mountain - **M**
  15 - 5 reps
  12 - 5 reps

- Cycle - **C**
  15 - 6 reps
  12 - 6 reps

- Monster Set - **MO**

Movements	Type of Set					Real				Intended		
Lower Body Movements	D	P	M	C	MO	Reps		Weight		Reps		Weight

10 Minutes   20 Minutes   30 Minutes

The Daily BBG Fitness Program

Body Parts: ....

Real Date	Real Time	Intended Date	Intended Time by God
	.... A.M./P.M.		.... A.M./P.M.

Types of Sets

•Decline - **D**	•Mountain - **M**	•Cycle - **C**
15 - 5 reps	15 - 5 reps	15 - 6 reps
12 - 5 reps	12 - 5 reps	12 - 6 reps
•Pause - **P**		•Monster Set - **MO**
12 - 0 reps		
12 - 0 reps		

Legs:
Upper Body:

Movements

Upper-Body Movements	Type of Set					Real		Intended	
	D	P	M	C	MO	Reps	Weight	Reps	Weight

30 Minutes   20 Minutes   10 Minutes

Generalized Personal Time Chart

MORNING/AFTERNOON

Time:	Time:	Time:	Time:	Time:
Life:	Life:	Life:	Life:	Life:

AFTERNOON/EVENING

Time:	Time:	Time:	Time:	Time:
Life:	Life:	Life:	Life:	Life:

(SYL) (SYL) (SYL) (SYL)

SOLID YELLOW LINE (SYL)

Personal Time Chart

Morning / Afternoon

Time:	Time:	Time:	Time:
Life:	Life:	Life:	Life:
Missionary Work:	Missionary Work:	Missionary Work:	Missionary Work:
Prosperity Time:	Prosperity Time:	Prosperity Time:	Prosperity Time:

Afternoon / Evening

Time:	Time:	Time:	Time:
Life:	Life:	Life:	Life:
Missionary Work:	Missionary Work:	Missionary Work:	Missionary Work:
Prosperity Time:	Prosperity Time:	Prosperity Time:	Prosperity Time:

(SYL)   (SYL)   (SYL)   (SYL)

(SYL)

SOLID YELLOW LINE (SYL)

About the Author

Dr. Sheri Lerner owned one of the largest woman-owned chiropractic clinics in the world, located in Allentown, Pennsylvania. In the summer of 2004 she opened her second clinic in Celebration, Florida, which is the first of its kind in the world-famous city.

Dr. Lerner also works with the Body by God organization and runs the spouses' program for Teach the World About Chiropractic, an international consulting, product, and seminar firm for a worldwide network of chiropractors. She has also run the Lehigh Valley Health and Wellness Foundation for Lifechurch, a church in Allentown. She organizes and speaks at community outreach seminars, pastors' conferences, health fairs, women's groups, and other health and wellness related events.

Dr. Lerner also knows firsthand about developing strong time management, managing stress, eating healthy, and forming exercise habits. Because of this she was able to bounce back after her pregnancy and will help you to as well.

She and her husband, Dr. Ben Lerner, enjoy their beautiful daughter, Nicole, and Ben's son, Skylar.

Acknowledgments

I want to say a special word of thanks to the Body by God providers throughout the world. They are my friends and the leaders in health-care in their communities. To learn more about them visit our Web site at http://www.thebodybygod.com/careproviders.html.